D0293623

S
STAMPED

A Gaia **Busy Person's** Guide

Aromatherapy

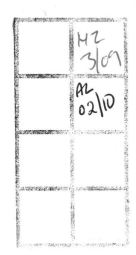

H2
3/09

AZ
02/10

Bristol Library Service

AN 2929279 4

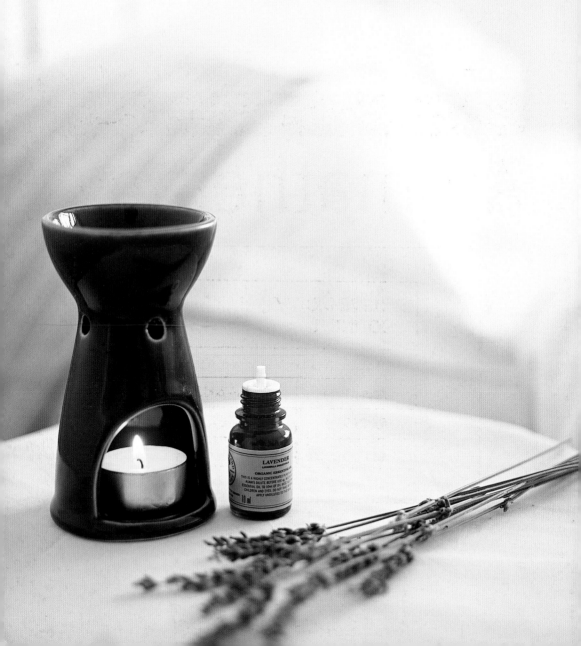

A Gaia **Busy Person's** Guide

Aromatherapy

Simple routines for home, work, & travel

BRISTOL CITY COUNCIL	
Askews	05-Jul-2005
615.3219	£9.99

Sarah Dean

Gaia Books

A Gaia Original

Books from Gaia celebrate the vision of Gaia, the self-sustaining living earth, and seek to help its readers live in greater personal and planetary harmony.

Editor	Jonathan Hilton
Design	Peggy Sadler
Editorial Direction	Jo Godfrey Wood
Art Direction	Patrick Nugent
Production	Louise Hall
Photography	Ruth Jenkinson
Proofreading and Index	Kathie Gill
Editorial consultant	Daphne Roubini MAR IFPA

Copyright © 2005 Gaia Books,
an imprint of Octopus Publishing Group,
2–4 Heron Quays, London, E14 4JP

Text copyright © 2005 Sarah Dean

The right of Sarah Dean to be identified as the author of this work has been asserted in accordance with Sections 77 and 78 of the Copyright, Designs and Patents Act 1988, United Kingdom. All rights reserved including the right of reproduction in whole or in part in any form.

First published in the United Kingdom in 2005 by Gaia Books Ltd

ISBN 1-85675-212-7
EAN 9 781856 752121

A catalogue record of this book is available from the British Library.

Printed and bound in China

10 9 8 7 6 5 4 3 2 1

Contents

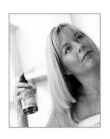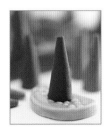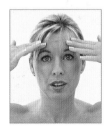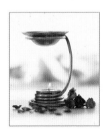

Using this book

This book is designed to offer you a comprehensive range of aromatherapy techniques in a format that is not only easy to use, but also reflects the needs of a modern, busy lifestyle.

From the moment you wake up, aromatherapy can be your companion throughout the rest of the day. Learn how to use essential oils for a vital boost in the morning, to stay alert during a long afternoon meeting, to soothe a tension headache, to re-energize yourself in preparation for an evening out, or to unwind and de-stress when staying in. Alternatively, just dip into this book whenever you need an immediate natural remedy – you can treat earache, paper cuts, and colds, or enjoy some truly nurturing essential oil recipes for room sprays, perfumed sheets, delicious-smelling hair, and aroma-facials.

Basic techniques, from how to smell an oil correctly to giving mini-massages, are all included and all geared totally to your environment. When an aromatherapy burner or a massage just isn't a practical proposition – when you are on the move, for example, or at work – this book offers you great alternatives, from essential oil pendants to aromatherapy stones and home-made vaporizers.

Chapter 1 explains the principles of aromatherapy and all the basic techniques, including massage strokes. Morning remedies appear in Chapter 2, along with an essential oil "capsule kit" to meet your daily needs; Chapter 3 comes with great travel ideas, plus remedies for jet lag, travel sickness, and commuter stress. In Chapter 4 are the many ways you can make

your working life less of a pain – literally – and enjoy
better concentration and energy, before unwinding at
the end of the day with the relaxation recipes and
techniques in Chapter 5. In order to find out more
about the individual oils that are used in
aromatherapy, refer to Chapter 6, which contains a
directory of essential oils. This section also includes
information on the carrier, or base, oils you will need
to blend with the essential oils used for massage.

THE SYMBOLS DECODED

*In the essential oil profiles on pages 120–37, the following symbols are displayed as a quick
guide to the relevant application of each oil:*

Use in an essential oil burner – or a diffuser or vaporizer (see pages 24–7).

Use in the bath (see page 29).

Use in massage, diluted in a carrier, or base, oil (see pages 30–2).

*Use for inhalation, by smelling from the bottle held at chin level (see page 25), added to
a bowl of water – cover your head with towels and inhale (see page 28), or added to a cup
of hot water.*

*Use in a mister bottle on hair or skin (see page 27). Note that all the essential oils listed
can be used in a mister bottle as a room spray, but only those that carry this symbol can
be used on skin or hair.*

Use as a perfume (see page 33).

Safety guidelines

This book serves as an introduction to aromatherapy and the use of essential oils, and it is not intended as a substitute for medical attention from a health professional. Before attempting to treat more serious physical or emotional conditions, please consult a professional aromatherapist, medical herbalist, or medical doctor. Essential oils should not be used at home to treat acute medical or psychological problems. Any application of the ideas and information contained in this book are at the reader's sole discretion and responsibility.

It is essential to adhere to the following guidelines:

- Don't exceed the recommended quantities of oils given in the recipes throughout this book. Using more oil does not mean that the recipe will be any more effective, and, indeed, exceeding the stated quantities can be dangerous.
- Never take essential oils internally – essential oils are for external use only. Some of the oils are toxic if taken internally.
- Generally, never apply essential oils directly to the skin or hair, unless specified (lavender and tea tree oil may sometimes be applied undiluted). Always dilute essential oils in a carrier, or base, oil, or in water if they are intended for misting.
- After using some essential oils, wait for between four and six hours before going out in the sun or having laser hair treatment, as they can make the skin photosensitive and will therefore cause irritation.

The oils to be aware of in this respect are bergamot, orange, grapefruit, and lemon grass.
■ Do not self-treat with essential oils if you are pregnant (see below).

IF YOU ARE PREGNANT

This book is not aimed at the treatment of babies or children, or for use during pregnancy. It is not recommended that pregnant or breastfeeding women self-treat with any essential oil, apart from dilute rose and geranium, which are considered safe throughout all stages of pregnancy.

However, if you are pregnant it, is recommended that you seek your doctor's approval and have treatment only from a qualified aromatherapist before using any essential oil.

Note that the cautions for pregnancy given in the essential oil profiles are included as an additional warning against using oils that may potentially be harmful during pregnancy.

OTHER CAUTIONS

If you suffer from epilepsy, high blood pressure, deep-vein thrombosis, varicose veins, or any other significant medical condition, please consult your doctor, a professional aromatherapist, or medical herbalist. If you are taking homeopathic remedies, do not use peppermint or eucalyptus essential oils. Ask your homeopath for advice on combining aromatherapy and homeopathy.

Some essential oils can have quite a dramatic effect on you physically and, therefore, may affect any long-term medication you are taking. Consult your doctor or a professional aromatherapist if this applies to you.

Introduction

In using aromatherapy as a part of your daily routine you are following an age-old tradition: in ancient Egypt, resins were burned in the morning, myrrh at noon, and kyphi at sunset as an offering to the sun god Ra. Kyphi, a famous blend of 16 or so essential oils, including myrrh and juniper, was thought to heighten the spiritual awareness of the priests. Used for healing and magical rites, essential oils were also an intrinsic part of the ritual of mummification. When Tutankhamen's tomb was opened in 1922, pots within the sarcophagus were found to contain precious myrrh and frankincense.

We practise aromatherapy instinctively, just as our ancestors did. The sense of smell acts as one of our greatest health protectors, an early-warning system against unpleasant or harmful substances. In fact, scent was, and still is, so vital to our survival that the millions of scent-detecting nerve-ending cells in our nose are renewed every 28 days – equivalent to a full lunar cycle, the natural rhythm of life.

Essential oils were used up to 6,000 years ago in the ancient civilizations of India, China, Greece, and Italy, although aromatherapy was formalized only within the last century. The word "aromatherapy" was first coined in 1928 by French chemist Dr René-Maurice Gattefossé (1881–1950); and aroma cosmetology – the practice of aromatherapy in health and beauty – was pioneered by French biochemist Marguerite Maury (1895–1968), who set up clinics in England, Paris, and Switzerland. Aromatherapy is now established in Europe, Australia, New Zealand, and America.

AN ANCIENT EGYPTIAN ELIXIR TO INSPIRE THE LOVE OF ALL WOMEN
Rose oil
Crushed rose petals
The oxyrhynchus, a fish of the Nile, burned to charcoal

The charcoal was ground to dust and mixed with the rose oil, then anointed on the man's head; and all women would desire him.

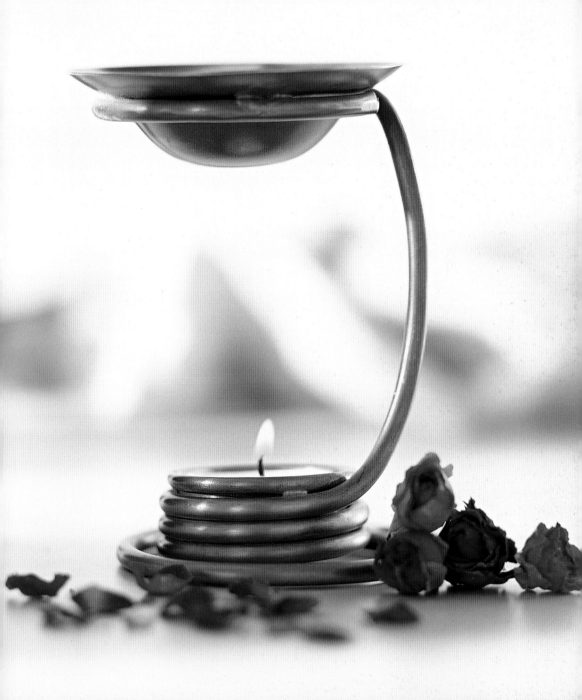

The gift of aromatherapy

Aromatherapy means "treatment using scents". Using essential oils is an effective way to experience sensational aromas and benefit from their healing properties – the pure essence of a plant in a tiny bottle you can carry with you anywhere.

Aromatherapy is one of the most popular forms of complementary medicine. The "aroma" in the therapy is the fragrant essence, or essential oil, secreted by the cells of plants and trees. Essential oils act on the mind and the body simultaneously via the skin and olfactory system (the sense of smell) to balance and heal, making it an ideal, gentle medicine that is not only therapeutic, but also enjoyable.

Essential oils have been used for thousands of years for religious and magical rituals, embalming, and healing. Dr René-Maurice Gattefossé, the French chemist who coined the term "aromatherapy", discovered one of the properties of lavender oil when he accidentally burned his hand in his laboratory and inadvertently applied the oil to the wound – the lavender soothed the pain, speeded the healing, and prevented scarring. Today, medical doctors and aromatherapists continue to research these amazing elixirs of life as they grow ever-more popular as an integral part of modern living.

It is easy to treat yourself using essential oils. This chapter explains how to buy and keep your oils, and it describes all the techniques you will need to introduce essential oils into your life. From aromatherapy massage to aromatic baths, here's how to find balance, better energy, more concentration … and less stress.

What are essential oils?

An essential oil is usually the active ingredient, or life force, of a plant or tree. Present in varying quantities in the leaf, stem, flower, bark, sap, heartwood, root, and fruit peel, the oil is generally responsible for a plant's fragrance, however subtle or potent.

Essential oils are considered to be so special because some have been found to contain phyto-hormones, or plant hormones, which can affect our bodies' systems, just as our own hormones can control heart rate, body temperature, appetite, or sleep patterns, for example. And since plant fragrances are designed to attract pollinators, essential oils have also been likened to human pheromones – a type of hormone responsible for our personal body scent, or "chemistry", that stirs up a reaction, such as sexual attraction or a sense of calm, in others.

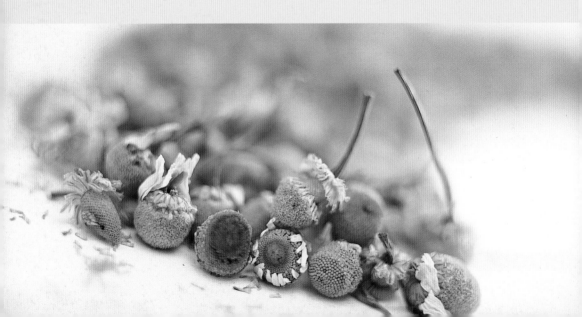

As well as seducing pollinators, a plant's essential oils act to deter leaf-munchers and other destructive pests. Allelopathy, or the study of the effect of one plant's chemistry on another, describes the way in which some plants even talk to each other. Plants and trees, such as the sunflower, alfalfa, eucalyptus, and walnut, can tell others to back off by using their special chemistry as an invisible weapon to deplete the growth of any encroaching competitors. Chamomile, conversely, is known as the "plants' physician", because it is said actively to encourage the health of any other plant it grows beside.

It is no surprise, therefore, to learn that these powerful oils have complex chemical structures. An essential oil is thought to contain at least 100 individual components, which can have varying actions – calming aldehydes or energizing alcohols and phenols, for example – all working together in synergy: in other words, producing a result that is greater than the sum of the parts.

It is virtually impossible to create a perfect synthetic version of an essential oil, because the imitation cannot contain the life force that is exclusive to the original. In addition, the full constituents of some essential oils, such as rose, are not known, making them even harder to mimic artificially.

TIMES OF DAY TO PICK HERBS AND FLOWERS

The Greek botanist and physician Pedanius Dioscorides (c.40–90 CE) found that the oil yield of a plant, and therefore its scent, fluctuates according to the time of day. As the essential oil cells in the plant change throughout the day, sometimes they possess a higher percentage of oil and so smell more enticing. On summer evenings the scent of flowers, such as honeysuckle, for example, become exceptionally strong and heady. Naturally, plants are harvested when their oil content is highest:

- *Lavender has more oil and scent between 10am and 4pm.*
- *Jasmine has most oil and scent at night.*
- *Rose has more oil before 10am.*

How essential oils work

Essential oils work on the mind and body simultaneously, and so we respond to their presence both physically and psychologically. And this reaction begins when we smell an essential oil's aroma or absorb it through our skin, which is the body's largest organ.

When we inhale an essential oil, the molecules it contains enter our lungs and from there pass into the bloodstream. Here they interact with the hormones and enzymes in the blood to affect our entire body chemistry. The molecules affect our body systems, too, calming or stimulating the immune system, digestion, nervous system, the endocrine/genito-urinary system, and skin, for example. In addition, the smell stimulates the brain's limbic system (the home of our emotions and memories), which triggers feelings and so affects our mood.

When you apply an essential oil to your skin (with the exception of tea tree and lavender, all oils are diluted with a carrier or base oil before use), the oil molecules are so small that they penetrate the skin and readily enter the circulation. Later, they are easily excreted from the body – usually within 6–14 hours – leaving no toxic residue.

Generally, all essential oils are antiseptic and usually specialize in treating particular types of infection – viral, bacterial, fungal, and parasitical. Some oils and herbs, such as lavender and ginseng, act in the body in a specific way. Known as adaptogens, they support the function of the adrenal glands to help the body adapt to and deal with stress.

So there is much more to aromatherapy than a few nice scents – essential oils have an intelligent physical and psychological effect on the body, acting therapeutically to help calm, energize, and heal.

AROMA AND MEMORY
In 1989 Professor Joseph LeDoux at the Center for Neural Science at New York University in the United States suggested that the amygdala, which is part of the limbic system – the primal brain responsible for motivation and memory – was concerned with storing the memories of frightening experiences. Stimulating the amygdala through scent, therefore, could be like using a key to unlock traumatic memories. This may be one of the reasons why the renowned aromatherapist Valerie Ann Worwood describes essential oils as "the little keys that can unlock our physical and mental mechanisms".

Of course smell is just one route to the past. See an old photograph, hear that tune and you will be immediately transported back to another time; all our senses may act as time machines in certain situations. Interestingly, one discussion website is debating the use of aroma under examination conditions. Unable to carry the academic equivalent of the old photograph or piece of music into the examination hall, the site author ponders if you could legitimately take in an essential oil or other fragrance. Because aroma can trigger memory, if one revised while burning basil oil, for example, and then later inhaled that same oil, would the required information come flooding back

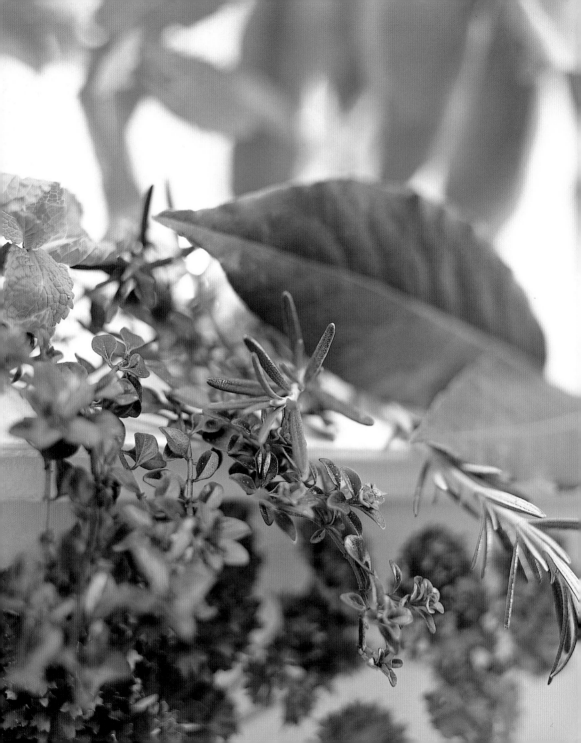

on call? This type of learning is known as "context-dependent", and uses an association, which may be aural, oral, visual, tactile, or olfactory, to encourage memory. Thankfully, the webmaster does add a cautionary postscript that using essential oils in this way "is no substitute for hard work".

Try rosemary oil for improving your memory, and basil, which is renowned for stimulating the mind and is perfect for concentration (see pages 129 and 127).

AROMA-BONDING

How is it that we can adore one fragrance – and even regard it as part of our identity – but later, turn up our noses at it? Once loyal to Coco Chanel, you fall hopelessly for the new Gucci fragrance, as your old, too-sweet perfume now does nothing for you. Yet it's not all about marketing, which can take you to the perfume counter, after all, but can't make you buy. You have to love the aroma.

Our aroma preferences shift because our bodies change as we age. As we grow older hormone levels alter, which has a great impact on our sense of smell. The change in oestrogen levels during pregnancy, for example, causes enhanced sensitivity particularly toward distinctive aromas, such as coffee, perfume, and cooking meat, often resulting in an aversion to some smells that were once loved or at least tolerated. After the menopause, when oestrogen levels drop, the woman's sense of smell changes once more as a whole new range of fragrances becomes attractive for the first time – a wonderfully unique reflection of ourselves as we evolve.

How to choose oils

Choosing organic essential oils means that the oil you buy is unadulterated and contains no synthetic additives, so its purity is guaranteed. Alternatively, choose a good-quality non-organic essential oil – one that has not been extracted using solvents, if possible. Oils produced by solvent extraction, which are known as "absolutes", do not contain as much therapeutic value.

Essential oils are obtained by steam distillation, expression, solvent extraction, and pressurized gas extraction. Steam distillation is the most common method of extraction – hot steam is passed through the plant parts to collect the essential oils, after which the steam is condensed and the oil separated from the water. The result is pure essential oil, and its by-product is floral water, such as lavender water or rose water. Expression – pressing and grinding fruit rinds – suits many citrus-type plants, such as grapefruit and lemon.

"Organic" does not always mean "best", so don't worry if you cannot always buy organic products. In some cases, oils from countries such as India may not receive organic certification due to a lack of information regarding the oil's origins, rather than because the product is substandard in any way. However, with the organic product the smell can be more delicious than that from a non-organic oil, and it can also have more "life force". Whichever oils you choose, be guided by your natural preference. Gently waft the bottle under your nose, at chin level, allowing the oil molecules to react with the air – sniffing the bottle directly could be overpowering (see Smelling an oil, page 25). If you like an oil, it follows that you will enjoy using it; if you feel duty-bound to use it because it is supposed to be good for your particular ailment but you hate the aroma, don't buy it. It is your body's way of telling you to choose something else.

When choosing essential oils the most crucial thing to make sure of is that they are genuine products. After you have checked the label, look for the price, which usually reflects the cost of extraction (see also page 22).

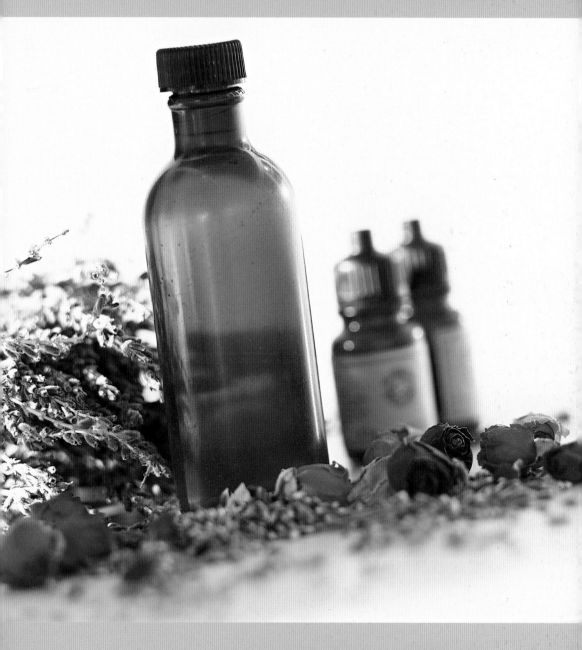

THE COST OF ESSENTIAL OILS

Below is a list of relative costs of essential oils commonly used and profiled in this book (see pages 120–37). Bear in mind that if you want to buy organic oils they are usually more expensive, and so will push some of the traditionally cheaper oils into the mid-range category. You may find that the cost of good-quality essential oils varies depending on the season.

Lower cost	Medium cost	High cost
Clove	Basil	Frankincense
Eucalyptus	Bergamot	Jasmine
Grapefruit	Cedarwood	Neroli
Lavender	Chamomile	Rose
Lemon	Clary sage	Sandalwood
Peppermint	Geranium	
Patchouli	Ginger	
Pine	Juniper	
Rosemary	Thyme	
Tea tree	Ylang ylang	

Storing oils

Store essential oils in airtight, dark containers away from sunlight. Don't leave the tops off the bottles or allow the oils to heat up, as this not only affects their qualities, but also allows them to evaporate needlessly. Provided that they are properly stored, most oils will last a few years.

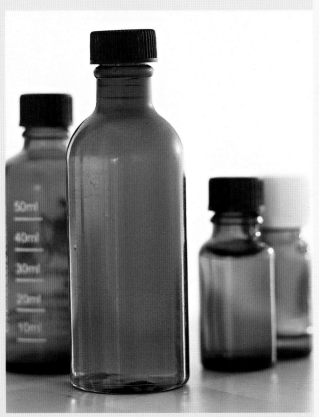

CHOOSING CARRIER OILS

For massage, you will need to dilute essential oils in a base, or carrier, oil, such as almond or grapeseed (see the chart on page 139 for a list of suggested oils). Opt for natural vegetable, nut, or seed oils – don't use mineral oil, such as baby oil, as it will not penetrate the skin effectively. Carrier oils will usually last up to two years, but again use your nose to guide you and never use an oil that smells even slightly bitter or unpleasant. This is a sure sign of deterioration.

Basic techniques

Here's how to use your essential oils. Bear in mind that some oils are not suitable for certain conditions or methods of application – see the essential oil profiles on pages 120-37 and the safety guidelines on pages 8–9.

OIL BURNERS

Also known as fragrancers, aromatherapy oil burners work by heating a few drops of oil in a water bowl set above a tea-light candle. An oil burner is a good investment as it's one of the easiest ways to benefit from an essential oil's perfume and mild therapeutic effect, and try out combinations of oils without applying them to your skin.

To use the burner, add essential oils to the water in the bowl and light the candle. Watch for a few minutes until you see a little mist or steam rise from the water – this mist carries the essential oils into the room. Then blow out the candle. You don't need to keep the candle burning to keep the aroma going. Remember never to leave a lit burner unattended.

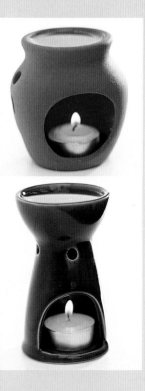

SMELLING AN OIL
To smell an oil, waft the open bottle under your nose, moving it from the right to the left at about chin height while you gently inhale. Don't sniff or use the bottle like an inhaler – this does not make the aroma more potent, and could be dangerous with oils that have overpowering aromas.

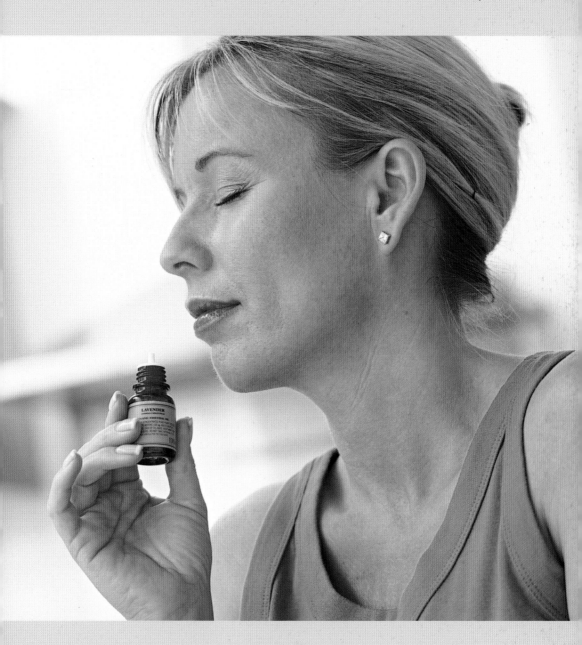

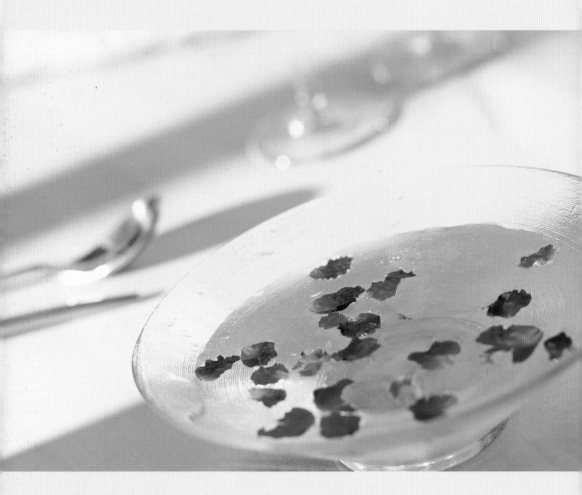

THAI TABLE OFFERING

For a romantic dinner setting, create a Thai table offering using a sweet and spicy combination, such as geranium and ginger. Fill a glass bowl with warm water and flower petals, such as those from roses or geraniums.

To the water, add:
3 drops geranium essential oil
1 drop ginger essential oil

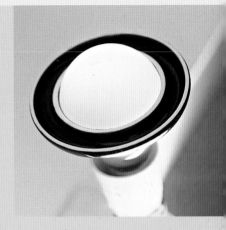

RING BURNERS

Aromatic ring burners, typically made of porcelain, terracotta, or aluminium, are designed to rest around the glass envelope of a light bulb so that the heat from the bulb stimulates the release of the scent.

VAPORIZERS AND DIFFUSERS

Vaporizers emit steam that carries the essential oil, whereas diffusers spray a fine mist of cold essential oil into the room. Some people prefer to use diffusers rather than vaporizers or burners, because diffusers do not use heat and so the molecular structure of the essential oil remains unchanged.

MISTING

You can mist with essential oils and flower waters (see page 51). To mist with essential oil, fill a mister bottle with water and add your oils (see page 50 for recipes), and then shake and spray. Depending on which oils you use, you can mist your hair, clothes, or face – but always close your eyes and avoid the eye area – along with your home and workspace.

QUICK METHOD

To purify the air in your home or office, add a few drops of essential oil to a small bowl of water placed on or near a warm radiator. Try citrus oils, such as grapefruit, lemon, or neroli, for an uplifting ambience.

INHALATIONS

Inhalation sounds like something your aunty did during the war years at the first hint of a cold, but inhalation – "inhaling" steam over a bowl of hot water under a tent of towels – is also great for your skin. As you breathe in the therapeutic oils, the steam acts to open up the pores and release the impurities. Make sure the steam is not too hot – hotter is not necessarily better, and overly hot steam can cause broken capillaries on the cheeks and irritate sensitive skin. To help a cold, add a few drops of eucalyptus, peppermint, or pine oil (see page 47 for more recipes).

SAUNAS

Using oils in a sauna is a great way to enjoy the benefits of aromatherapy. If you are not lucky enough to have access to a private sauna, you will need to belong to a health club that permits the use of essential oils.

Add a few drops of essential oils to the hot coals, or take a massage oil you have prepared earlier and rub it into your skin as soon as you enter the sauna. As you sit or lie down on a towel, the heat will help your skin absorb the oil as the aroma intensifies.

For a peaceful vibe, try sandalwood or rose essential oils, or, for a cheaper option, choose sweet-smelling palma rosa.

QUICK METHOD
Add a few drops of essential oil to a cup of hot water and inhale the aroma. Remember not to leave the concoction on your desk, where you might later mistake it for a cup of water and drink it. Empty the cup straight after use.

WOOD FIRES

Add your chosen oils to the wood a few hours or so before lighting the fire. In this way, the oils sink into the wood itself. You can also pick aromatic herbs from your garden for burning in an open fire – rosemary, lavender, and sage smell divine. Sage is used traditionally in space-clearing, or "smudging", rituals (see pages 82–5), in which herb smoke is wafted around a room to purify negative energy.

BATHS

This is one of the most popular ways to enjoy aromatherapy. Run a bath, then add a few drops of your chosen oils (don't add the oils while the taps are running, as the oil will evaporate before the benefits can be enjoyed). If you use bubble bath, the essential oil becomes caught in the bubbles and can't be properly dispersed. Disperse the oil by waving your hand rapidly over the surface of the water. Oils suitable for bathing include geranium (wonderful for lifting your spirits in the morning) and lavender (a great soporific before going to bed).

MASSAGE

Aromatherapists use a carrier, or base, oil, in which essential oils are diluted before being massaged into the skin. On these pages, and on page 32, are four principal massage strokes, each with an application.

Effleurage

This gliding stroke smoothes the oil over the skin, and is used to begin and end a massage. Effleurage boosts the circulation, improves the lymph flow, and relaxes the muscles.

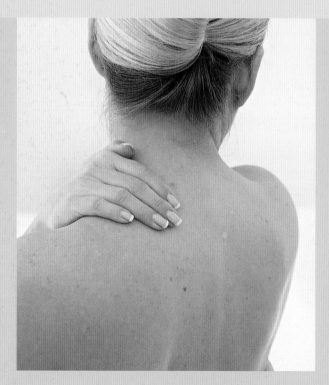

SHOULDER TENSION
Use your whole hand, keeping the pressure even, as you sweep over the ridge of your shoulder. Oils for tense muscles include lavender, rosemary, and chamomile (see pages 120, 129, and 121).

Petrissage
Petrissage describes kneading and rolling strokes that stimulate deep tissue and, like effleurage, get the circulation and lymph going.

Friction
Friction describes vigorous, circular strokes often used to stimulate tight areas of the back.

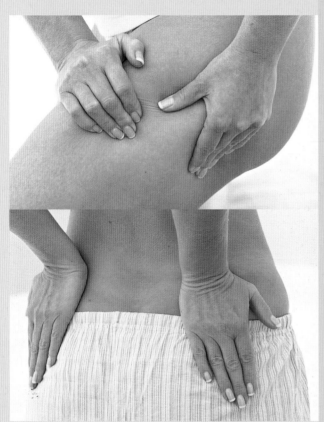

NOTE
This is a simple guide only – for detailed massage information, consult a dedicated massage manual.

CELLULITE
Imagine that you are gently kneading bread – with one hand, take hold of the flesh between your fingers and thumb, then release and repeat with the other hand in a continuous motion. Work upward, toward the heart, with a hand-over-hand movement. Essential oils that may help reduce cellulite include juniper and grapefruit (see pages 131 and 136.

LOWER BACK TENSION
Use both palms at the same time, each making symmetrical circles. As for shoulder tension (see opposite), oils such as lavender, rosemary, and chamomile can help muscle tension (see pages 120, 129, and 121).

Finger pressure

Finger pressure uses one or two fingers to release deep
tension in a small area, such as around the mouth.

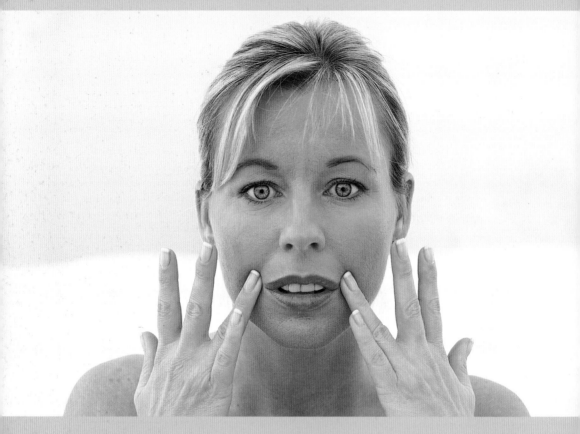

LAUGHTER LINES
*Rotate your ring fingers in small circles as you work upward
from the mouth toward the side of the nose. Oils that may
help guard against laughter lines include patchouli, neroli,
and chamomile (see pages 132 and 121).*

HAND CREAMS AND OILS

You can, of course, make natural hand creams, but an easier way to make the most of your essential oils when you don't have too much time is to add them to a perfume-free hand cream or a carrier oil, such as almond or avocado for very dry skin (see page 139).

COMPRESSES

An aromatic compress can help headaches, sprains, and bruising – add essential oils to 2 cups of warm water, dip in a folded flannel, squeeze out the excess liquid, and lay the flannel over the area you need to treat.

PERFUMES

Making perfume is a subject in itself, but making your own simple scents need not be complicated. To wear your favourite essential oil as a perfume, follow this basic recipe as a rule of thumb. Bear in mind, however, that the number of drops can vary depending on the oil used (see right):

3 drops essential oil
1 teaspoon carrier oil

Blend the essential oil and the carrier oil together and dab it on the usual perfume hot-spots – on the inside of the wrists and behind the ears.

WHAT'S IN A DROP?

In aromatherapy, essential oils are measured in drops – but not all drops are equal. Less-viscous oils have larger drops because they run more freely – these include citrus oils, such as lemon, bergamot, and grapefruit. Thicker, viscous oils, such as sandalwood, have a smaller drop size, so always watch the drop size when measuring oils to ensure accurate quantities.

CHAPTER TWO

Start your day with aromatherapy

How you feel when you wake up often sets

the mood for the day ahead. With aromatherapy,

you can help programme your mind and body to

feel good as soon as you stir, and help you feel

energized and positive as you meet the

challenges that each morning brings.

When you are semi-conscious – in that drowsy half-sleep state before you fully surface – your sense of smell is particularly sensitive. Even a subtle fragrance from the previous evening can ease you into wakefulness, from the perfume on your wrist to the lingering fragrance of sandalwood from last night's oil burner. Take a few deep breaths as you stretch out in bed, inhaling through your nose and exhaling through your mouth. Breathing deeply boosts the flow of blood and oxygen in the body, helping to get you moving, and allows you to sense all the aromas around you. Don't forget to appreciate those scents you adore but often take for granted, because they, too, are aromatherapy at its simplest and perhaps most instinctive level: fresh-scented bed linen that reminds you of summer or a blast of fresh coffee and toast that leads your tentative limbs toward the kitchen.

Fill your waking moments with great aromas and you will benefit from the warm feelings they bring. This is because aromas with positive associations affect the brain – like chocolate stimulating the release of endorphins, the body's happiness chemicals.

In this chapter are creative ways to bring aromatherapy into your life, beginning with those precious seconds just after the alarm goes off.

Aromatherapy to start the day

Essential oils can help to lift your spirits as you start the day, and there are many ways in which to enjoy their aromas. From showering in your own aromatherapy "steam" room to simply smelling a dilute wake-up oil, aromatherapy can help you feel more grounded and less stressed, even when you have a frantic timetable ahead.

If you sleep well, you feel more rested and positive in the morning, so getting off to a good start often means a good night's rest. In the evening, you can use an aromatherapy stone, vaporizer, diffuser, or essential oil burner (see pages 24–9) to perfume your bedroom. Essential oils can help with insomnia and instil peace of mind, helping you to wake up worry free.

The recipe's title below comes from an anxiety that probably stems from childhood, having reached Sunday evening in a state of denial about all the homework still left to do before the morning. This tradition slides into adult life, too, as the sanctity of Sunday afternoon passes into evening panic about work the next day.

In the following recipe, the oils bergamot, sandalwood, and chamomile act as relaxants, and sandalwood is also said to encourage dreaming. Add the stated quantities to the water in the essential oil burner:

Sunday night calm
1 drop bergamot essential oil
2 drops sandalwood essential oil
1 drop chamomile essential oil

If you are using a burner to perfume your bedroom, allow the tea-light to burn for a few minutes until the oils mist (see page 24). If the room is cold you can let the tea-light burn for up to 20 minutes, but do not leave the burner unattended while it is lit. Blow out the candle and drift off into a deep, satisfying sleep. When you wake, you will inhale the subtle, calming ambience of the burned oils.

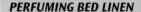

PERFUMING BED LINEN

You can add neat essential oils to your pillow, provided that they do not irritate your skin (see pages 8–9). Good oils to start with are lavender and chamomile. Sprinkle two or three drops of either oil onto a tissue and inhale gently, or sprinkle lavender onto the corners of your pillowcases.

For naturally perfumed sheets, dilute your chosen oils in half a pint of cold water and during the rinse cycle add it to the tray in your washing machine where you usually pour the washing liquid. Make sure that you use unscented washing liquid or powder so that the more delicate aroma of the oils is not overpowered.

Always choose essential oil aromas that you love; otherwise the fragrance will disrupt your sleep and potentially cause discomfort.

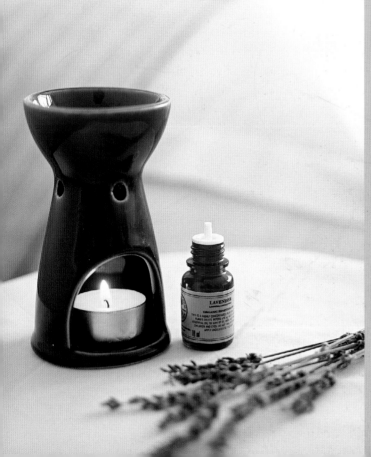

Oils to wake up with

Some essential oils will wake you up almost as quickly as the alarm clock. You can use these natural energizers in seconds as modern-day smelling salts, literally to bring you around, although in this case only from a sleepy state, rather than a fainting fit or an "attack of the vapours".

Bergamot, basil, and peppermint oils are great for early starts – just add a few drops of your chosen oil to a cup of hot water and inhale slowly, or drop the neat oil onto a tissue and hold it under your nose. If this is too intense for you, go for peppermint tea. Give yourself a few minutes to sip the infusion and inhale the scent as you gradually revive. If you can, avoid drinking coffee in the morning – it may act like rocket fuel to get you springing out of the front door, but the downside is that it will make you feel tense before the day has even begun. Go for herbal teas or warm water with lemon.

EIGHT WAYS TO ENERGIZE YOURSELF

The uplifting oils listed here have added benefits to help you deal with those weekday mornings. For a fuller list of the properties that are associated with each oil, see the essential oil profiles on pages 120–37.

Essential oil	Qualities
Bergamot	Calms stress and irritability, releases "stuck" energy
Basil	Awakens the mind
Geranium	A mood-enhancer; calms worry
Grapefruit	A detoxifying tonic
Lemon	Refreshes; promotes a sense of humour
Peppermint	A stimulant; eases headaches
Rosemary	Boosts the body into action; enhances memory
Thyme	Fights lethargy

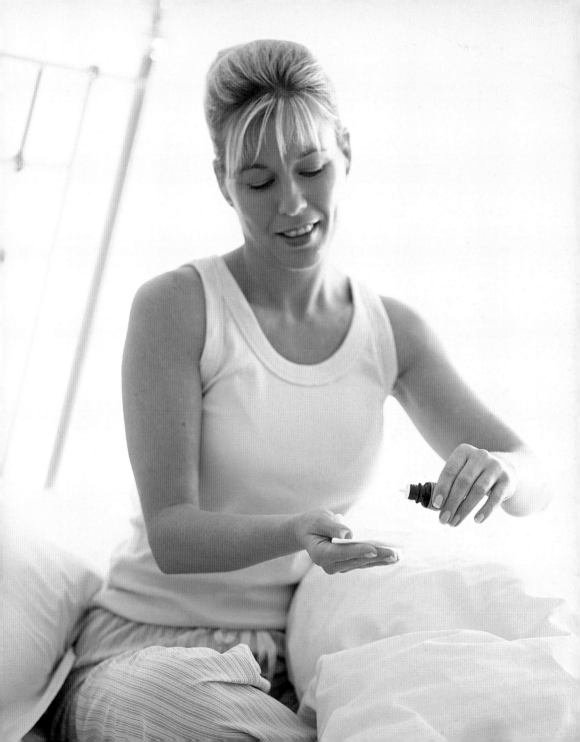

Aroma steam and shower

An aromatherapy "steam-shower" and scalp massage will revitalize your circulation, improving blood flow to the brain so that you will not only think better, you will also feel great. Combining the right essential oils in hot water in the hand basin, along with a little self-massage, takes only ten minutes or so, but the benefits will last throughout the day.

First, fill the hand basin with very hot water and add the essential oils (see below). Keep the bathroom door and the window closed and let the oils infuse for a few minutes so that the whole room fills with aromatic steam. Then take a hot shower, and try the head massage on page 42.

Steam blend for focused attitude

2 drops basil essential oil
2 drops bergamot essential oil

Basil and bergamot awaken the mind, ease tension, and help you prepare for a pressurized day.

Steam blend for vitality

2 drops lemon essential oil
2 drops rosemary essential oil

Lemon and rosemary refresh and invigorate, acting as an energy tonic.

Rosemary hair rinse

*To a jug of tepid water, add:
2 drops rosemary essential oil*

Rinsing the hair with dilute rosemary gives your hair shine and strength, stimulating the scalp.

Lemon deodorant

Add two drops of lemon essential oil to water in a mister bottle, shake well, and spray it on as an effective deodorant. Don't use it immediately after getting out of the bath or shower – instead, give your pores five minutes or so to close a little and so avoid possible skin irritation.

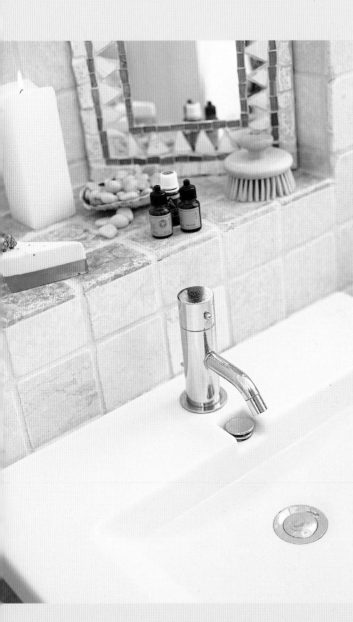

JUNIPER SCRUB FOR ACHES AND PAINS

Aromatherapy can help whenever you suffer from post-exercise stiffness. If a new gym workout means you have woken to tight or aching muscles, you can still treat yourself, even if you have only a few minutes in the morning. Stretch as soon as you get out of bed to get your muscles moving, then make up this aromatic scrub, which uses juniper essential oil to promote the elimination of the toxins that are responsible for muscle stiffness. You can prepare this the night before if you need to save time:

A handful of sea salt
15ml (1 tablespoon) almond oil, or enough to make the sea salt into a paste consistency
2 drops juniper essential oil

Mix well. Wet your body and apply the scrub to the areas of stiffness, massaging lightly in circular movements for a few minutes. Then shower off the scrub. Don't try this if you have dry or sensitive skin.

Aroma face and head massage

This type of head massage is beneficial any time, anywhere, and it makes no difference whether you massage wet or dry, or whether you use an essential oil blend or not. Massaging your scalp vigorously stimulates the circulation, helping you to wake up and feel more vital.

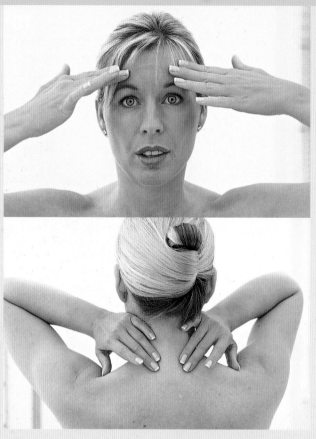

(01) Massage your scalp using circular movements with your fingertips. Continue circling, moving across the forehead from the middle of the forehead outward, toward the sides of the face.

(02) Circle your fingertips up the back of your neck, up to the occiput – the dip where the neck and back meet.
Then use your thumb and middle finger to gently pinch the bridge of your nose. This opens the bladder meridian, refreshing the whole body.

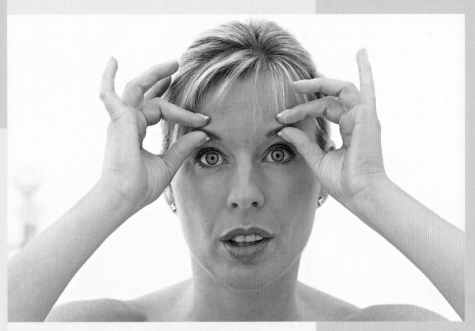

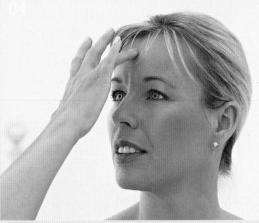

04

(03) *Continue this gentle pinching action outward from the bridge of your nose, moving along the ridge of both eyebrows.*

(04) *Exert steady pressure between your eyebrows (the third eye position), then press at the mid-point of your forehead, and thirdly at the "peak" of the hairline. To finish, gently tug at your hair to invigorate your scalp.*

Hangover rescue

In the morning we usually get a taste of what the day might bring, at least physically, such as the sniffle that forecasts a cold. Hangovers, however, those "accidental" consequences of late-night drinking, predict a day of painful reminders in the form of a crashing headache and some vague guilt about self-inflicted suffering. The only consolation is that a hangover does tend to improve as the day goes on, and by three o'clock it may, thankfully, have deserted you.

In the morning, when you have no time for a hangover, you can call on essential oils for help. Bear in mind that one hangover symptom is an extra sensitivity to aromas, so tread carefully with the oils listed on the right and only use them if you like them.

You can apply the blend to the pulse points – your wrists and temples – but one of the most effective ways to use the hangover formula is in a foot massage.

You can also add the neat oils to a basin- or sinkful of hot water, but omit the rose essential oil if you like, as it is expensive. If you are pressed for time, add the oils to a cup of hot water, gently inhaling the steam for a minute or so. However you choose to use the hangover formula, it's worth bottling it and taking it out with you so you can use it whenever you need to. Also remember to drink as much water as you can manage to alleviate the dehydration that comes from drinking alcohol, and for energy add a little honey to a herbal tea, such as peppermint, which is traditionally recommended for headaches.

HANGOVER FORMULA
Choose two oils from this list:

1 drop lemon essential oil
1 drop juniper essential oil
1 drop grapefruit essential oil
1 drop rose essential oil
1 drop peppermint essential oil

Dilute the two oils in 30ml (2 tablespoons) of carrier oil, such as grapeseed (see pages 138–9).

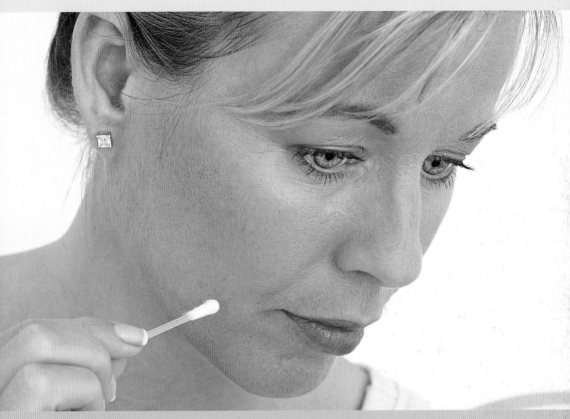

SPOT CHECK

If spots or cold sores are the first thing to greet you in the mirror, treat them with lavender or tea tree essential oils. Using a Q-tip (cotton bud), dab a little of the neat oil directly onto the spot or cold sore. All essential oils have antiseptic properties, but lavender and tea tree are renowned for spot and cold-sore treatment, particularly as they are usually the only two oils used neat on the skin.

Treating colds and boosting energy

Colds and flu have myriad symptoms, from low energy to fever, exhaustion, aches, sore throats, coughs, and colds. When you are not sure if a morning cough will turn into a full-blown cold but can't spend a day at home undisturbed just in case, use essential oils to ward off those flu-like feelings and boost your immunity.

To relieve the symptoms of a cold, choose one of the following oils, add a few drops to a cup of hot water, and gently inhale the steam. Or, add a few drops of your preferred oil to a tissue to smell: lavender, bergamot, eucalyptus, peppermint, pine, tea tree, ginger, sandalwood, or rosemary.

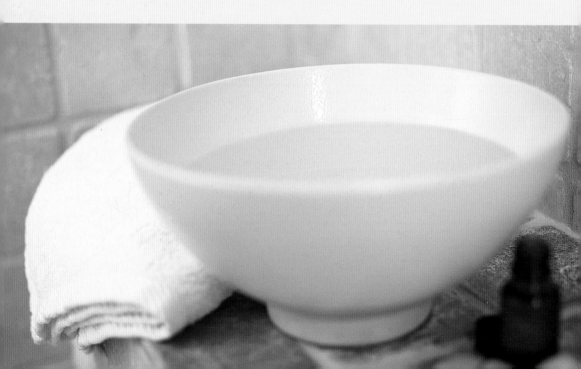

When you have more time, prepare an essential oil blend for colds using the recipe suggestions here and use them in steam inhalations, massage, baths, and in aromatherapy burners:

INHALATION FORMULA FOR COLDS
Add the following formula to a bowl of steaming water. Place a towel over your head and slowly inhale to take in the aroma.

Warming blend
2 drops eucalyptus globulus essential oil
1 drop tea tree essential oil
2 drops rosemary essential oil

Or

Cooling blend
2 drops lavender essential oil or eucalyptus citriodora
2 drops tea tree essential oil
1 drop lemon essential oil

HERBAL TEAS FOR A COLD
Try lemon and ginger tea with honey – use fresh root ginger, sliced and immersed in boiling water with a slice of lemon or a drop of fresh-squeezed lemon juice. Leave for five minutes or so before adding a teaspoon of honey to soothe a sore throat. For a head cold, try peppermint tea. You may also want to take the herbal supplement, echinacea. Some people find that it improves their immunity to coughs and colds.

MASSAGE AND BATHING BLENDS FOR A COLD
To use these blends, dilute in 45ml (3 tablespoons) of a carrier oil, such as almond or grapeseed.

Warming blend
1 drop ginger
1 drop eucalyptus globulus
1 drop tea tree
1 drop clary sage

Or

Cooling blend
1 drop peppermint
1 drop bergamot
1 drop frankincense
1 drop eucalyptus citriodora

Use the warming blend if you are feeling chilled, and the cooling blend if you are feeling hot and feverish.

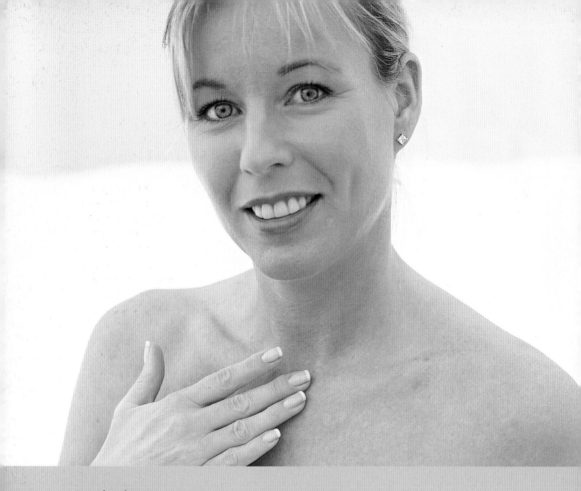

Cough mixture
You should never drink neat or even dilute essential oils, but you can still treat a hacking cough or cold using essential oils as an inhalation or as a massage. Ginger, for example, boosts the body's immunity and also has an anti-inflammatory action, relieving the aches and pains often associated with colds. Dilute the ginger and the other essential oils opposite in 30ml (2 tablespoons) of carrier oil and massage a little around the base of your throat and temples, (as shown above).

2 drops frankincense essential oil
1 drop ginger essential oil
1 drop eucalyptus essential oil

If you don't have time to prepare this formula, you can use lavender essential oil. Lavender has amazing antiseptic properties. Use this ratio for a beneficial blend:

2 drops lavender essential oil
2 teaspoons carrier oil

Dab the oil blend on your temples and down toward the jaw – this way you benefit from the aroma without applying the oil to the principal areas of the face.

Sore throat gargle
1 teaspoon sea salt
1 drop tea tree essential oil
1 drop lavender essential oil
1 drop clary sage essential oil

Add to tepid water, stir well, gargle, and spit out – do not swallow.

For mouth ulcers
1 teaspoon sea salt
1 drop tea tree essential oil
1 drop lavender essential oil

Add to tepid water, stir well, swish around your mouth, hold over the area of the ulcer, and spit out.

FOR CONJUNCTIVITIS
Take two chamomile tea bags, infuse them in a mug of hot water, and place a saucer on top and leave the liquid to go cold. With clean hands, squeeze out the tea bags and use them as eye masks. Then take two cotton cosmetic pads (make sure they are smooth, not fluffy, so that they don't irritate), immerse them in the cold tea, and use them to bathe your eyes. Wipe and repeat. You can keep the remaining cold tea in the refrigerator for later use.

Hair-omatherapy

Treating your hair to an aromatic mist in the morning is a great way to enjoy the therapeutic benefits of essential oils all day long. It's also a quick and easy way to neutralize those stale odours that surface in your consciousness as you begin to wake up. When you are drowsy, one sniff of your hair can trigger an olfactory flashback: from takeaway food to stale perfume and air pollution, the scent of your hair can tell a vivid story of the night before. Cigarette smoke, in particular, clings like a bad memory, and if you have no time to wash your hair before leaving home, the thought of enduring the day in a smoky aura can be enough to send you scurrying back under the duvet.

An effective solution is to mist your hair with dilute essential oils, a fragrant treatment that will not only freshen your hair naturally, but will also enhance your mood throughout the day.

It's simplicity itself to make your own blend. It will last for up to a week, provided that it is stored in an airtight dark-glass bottle away from sunlight. If you use a plastic mister bottle, decant any remaining solution into a dark-glass bottle straight after use. Or keep the mister bottle in the refrigerator – the dilute oils will keep for up to three days.

FOR FRESHENING HAIR
Grapefruit essential oil
Lemon essential oil

As well as banishing stale aromas, grapefruit and lemon help to fight fatigue.

FOR FRESHENING CLOTHES
Geranium essential oil
Lemon essential oil

Always spray in a fine mist and not on delicate fabrics.

WHAT YOU NEED
A mister bottle, preferably dark glass
A dark-glass bottle for storing leftover solution
Essential oils

Add a total of 4 drops of your chosen essence(s) to half a cup of water in a mister bottle. Shake and spray a fine mist 7 to 10cm (3 to 4in) from the hair, taking care not to get any in your eyes or on your face. Or add 4 or 5 drops of neat essential oil to a hairbrush (not directly on the hair) and brush it through.

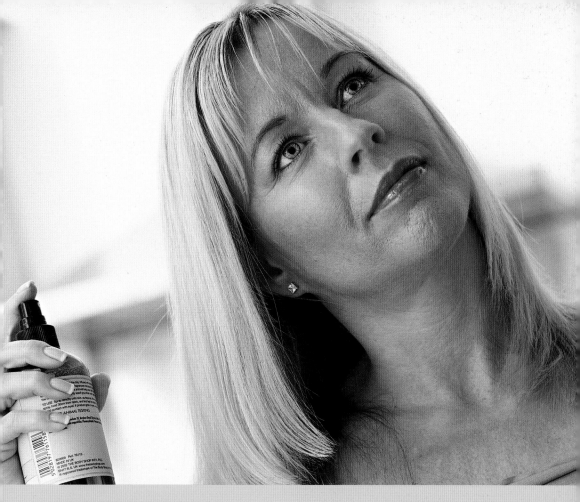

FLOWER WATER

As an alternative to using essential oils you can mist your hair with a flower water – try rose, orange, or lemon.

Flower waters are known by a variety of names, including hydrosols, hydroflorates, and distillates, and they are produced by steam-distilling plant materials.

Their properties are similar to those of essential oils, but since they are far less concentrated there is no need to add them to water before using them in a mister for your hair or clothes. Essential oils can also have a drying effect on the hair, so if your hair type is naturally prone to dryness then misting with a flower water may be a better alternative for you.

Capsule kit: the seven vital oils for your day

Regard the following oils as your essential daily kit. They have been selected because of the important benefits they confer – from basic first aid to better concentration and less stress.

Lavender: de-stressing, first aid for burns
It is soporific, relaxing, antiseptic, and helps to prevent blistering after a burn. It is one of the few essential oils that can be applied neat to the skin (see page 120).

Tea tree: natural antiseptic
Used to treat colds, insect bites and fungal infections, such as athlete's foot (see page 126).

Lemon: happiness
Another natural antiseptic, lemon eases irritability, is stimulating and refreshing, and is also thought to improve our sense of humour (see page 131).

Basil: for concentration
Fights fatigue and boosts concentration; helpful for studying or working late into the night (see page 127).

Geranium: uplifting, attraction
A natural mood-enhancer, geranium also helps ease depression. It helps people express their sensual side; in folklore, geranium was used to attract a lover (see page 123).

Peppermint: alertness, helps headaches

A great "wake-up" oil that also soothes headaches and helps indigestion (see page 122).

Chamomile: pain relief

De-stressing and anti-inflammatory, chamomile can help soothe period pain (see page 121).

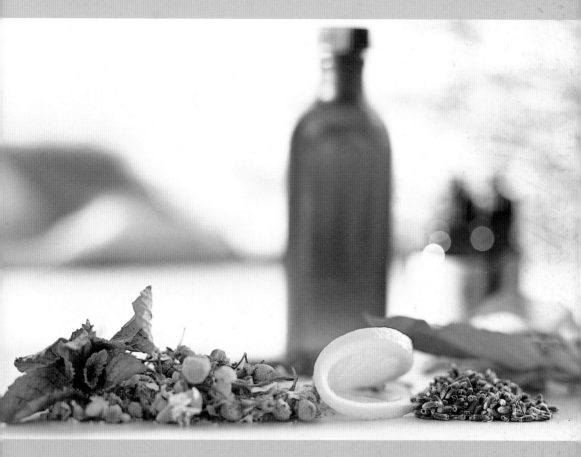

CHAPTER THREE

Aromatherapy on the move

Travelling can induce more potential stress than examinations, perhaps because we have so little control over our environment. From travel sickness to jet lag, packed trains to traffic gridlock, aromatherapy is the perfect remedy to help you when you are on the move.

A daily commute can bring about extreme reactions: road rage, total lethargy, stress, or sheer panic about being late. Travel further afield and a whole new raft of potential problems loom: the possibility of travel sickness, jet lag, check-in stress, and the aches and pains due to lugging around heavy suitcases are all enough to generate anxiety before your journey has even begun.

Travelling can make you feel more stressed and vulnerable than usual, particularly if you are commuting early in the morning before you are fully awake and properly alert. Travel stress can also deplete your immune system, because the intense worry it generates during a journey burns up your body's nutrient resources. Drink plenty of water if flying and avoid salty foods to prevent dehydration and water retention, which causes bloating and may trigger headaches. And give strong tea and coffee a miss, as the caffeine both of these drinks contain will make you feel even more tense.

There is also much you can do before you actually begin a journey to protect yourself while on the move. This chapter shows you how to use "grounding" essential oils, such as cedarwood and chamomile, to stave off travel stress and help you arrive at your destination feeling balanced and a little calmer. Because aromatherapy is easy to practise in your car, on a train, an aircraft, or simply while walking about, you will find that bottles of dilute essential oil are perfect travelling companions.

Get grounded

To get in good shape before you travel, always eat breakfast. Slow-to-medium energy-release foods will keep your blood sugar levels stable at least until mid-morning and keep you feeling more relaxed during a journey. Choose from wholemeal bread; boiled, scrambled, or poached eggs; porridge with linseed, or flaxseed (a natural superfood); fruit, such as banana, berries, and apple; and bio-yoghurts. Eat something for breakfast, no matter how little.

If you feel panicky or generally anxious in the morning before you leave home, gently inhale one of the following diluted oils to help you feel more grounded. First, however, take a few deep breaths – remember that the feeling will soon pass. Focus only on the rise and fall of your breathing as you relax. Add a few drops of the recommended oils to a cup of hot water and gently inhale the aroma. If you don't have any of these to hand, go for your favourite soothing oil (for more ideas, see pages 102–17).

Grounding oils
Cedarwood essential oil
Juniper essential oil
Bergamot essential oil

If you lack energy in the mornings, you can use oils to stimulate you and lift your spirits (see page 36). Whenever you feel listless or lethargic, pep yourself up with an energizing oil, such as bergamot or thyme – again, add a few drops of your chosen oil to a cup of hot water and inhale gently for a minute or so.

BREAKFAST BOOST
To get your day off to a good start make sure to eat a proper breakfast, such as yoghurt, porridge, muesli, and fruit.

USING BACH FLOWER REMEDIES
Bach Flower Remedies are flower essences suspended in alcohol that are designed specifically to work on the emotions. The most commonly used Bach remedy is Rescue Remedy™, which you can drop onto your tongue or dilute in water and drink whenever you need to calm down. If the sight of a packed train is enough to make you feel claustrophobic, stave off potential panic with Rescue Remedy™ and/or a little aromatherapy in the form of geranium essential oil inhaled from a tissue.

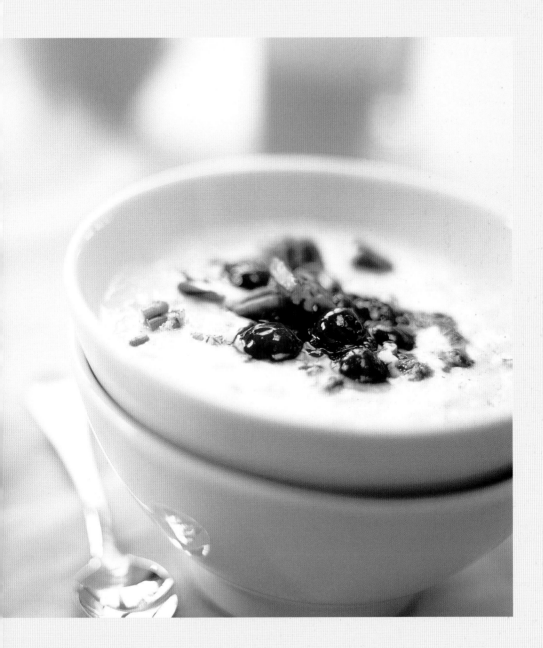

Travel sickness

Travel sickness is due to sensitivity of the inner ear, where we experience balance, and environmental factors, such as heat, motion, and general discomfort. We have yet to find the perfect remedy for travel sickness, and for decades alternative "cures" have been offered. Cars were once fitted with a length of conductive rubber that trailed along the ground when they moved, discharging the surplus static electricity thought to be responsible for travel sickness. No one knew at the time if this worked – the only certainty was that the conductive rubber prevented electric shocks from car doors. Today, people are experimenting with magnets as a way to prevent this inconvenient illness.

Travel sickness can be debilitating, and the worst cases often occur when you least expect them. If you usually suffer during long journeys by road, for example, it's easy to pre-empt illness by taking travel-sickness tablets before you set out (if they work for you). However, if you travel unexpectedly or hit bad weather conditions, turbulence on a plane or at sea, then sickness can ruin a trip. Carry dilute peppermint from the essential oil capsule kit (see pages 52–3) and you will be better prepared.

Smell ginger or peppermint oil diluted in one teaspoon of carrier oil, or gently inhale neat peppermint oil from the bottle, for on-the-spot travel-sickness relief. If you have access to refreshments on your journey, ask for chamomile or peppermint tea (or take your own tea bags), which also calms the stomach and aids digestion. In addition, you can:

ACUPRESSURE FOR TRAVEL SICKNESS
Locate the pressure point heart constrictor 6 on the inside of your wrist. It is found 5 cm (2 inches) up from the wrist crease – about three finger-widths – in line with the middle finger.

Massage this point using finger pressure to relieve the unpleasant symptoms.

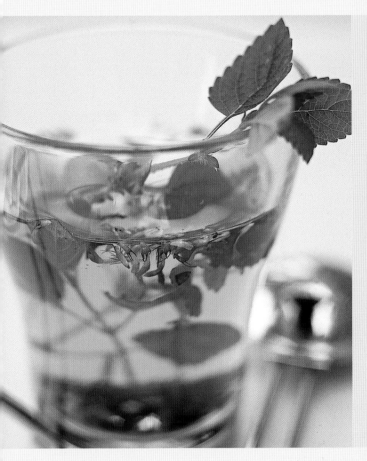

COMMERCIAL PEPPERMINT
Peppermint is cultivated commercially throughout Europe, the United States, and in Japan, and the essential oil from this plant finds its way into a wide range of products, including digestive tablets ideal for settling upset stomachs due to travel sickness.

- Focus on a distant, stationary object to counteract the feeling of motion.
- Stay as still as possible as you take several slow, deep, calming breaths.

Mini-meditation

Meditation with visualization can help to reduce some travel sickness and anxiety symptoms because it teaches you to switch your focus away from the immediate environment and mentally create positive sensations. Just being able to take action can be a stress release in itself, as worrying is often caused by feeling that you have no control over events. Travelling is a prime example of when you may feel particularly vulnerable to other people's decisions – when someone else is literally in the driving seat and you can do nothing about it, no matter how uncomfortable, late, or bored you may be.

REDUCING ANXIETY

■ *Before you set off, find a quiet place and sit cross-legged, as shown opposite. Close your eyes and take two or three deep, unhurried breaths, inhaling through your nose and exhaling through your mouth. Focus on this. Note when your breath rises and falls, and listen to its sound. Do this for several minutes.*

■ *As you breathe gently in and out, in your mind's eye see yourself as a small person stepping into a vast garden. Add the features of the landscape; choose whatever you would like to see – a river with pasture and cattle, wild flowers, a path to a windmill. Let your landscape take shape as you feel your body sink down into the earth. If you find this difficult, just return to focusing on the steady rise and fall of your breathing.*

■ *Now look closer at a single blade of grass, a stone, a flower – anything you choose to focus on in your landscape. Take in its detail as you continue to breathe, and feel the still sky above you. If you see flowers, smell their scents; if you wander closer to a stream, listen for the sound of the water. Use all your senses in your garden.*

■ *When you are ready, open your eyes.*

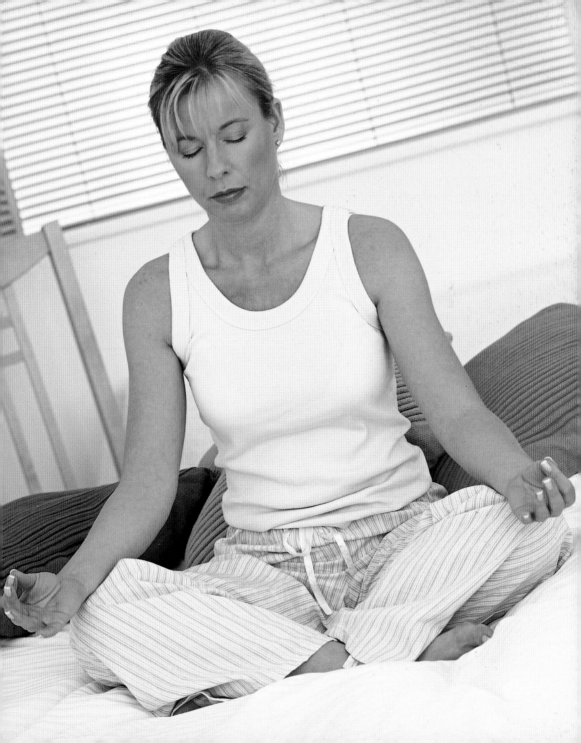

Portable remedies

On longer journeys, you can use aromatherapy to freshen up. Roll-ons, available from suppliers, are a convenient way to apply a ready-blended oil, and often there is a choice of energizing or calming formulas to select from. As well, keep an eye out for those tiny, stoppered oil phials that are designed to be worn as pendants – you can fill them with essential oil blends to inhale or dab on your wrists and neck whenever the need arises.

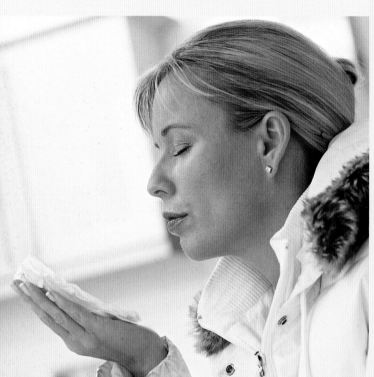

For long journeys
Measure a teaspoon of carrier oil, such as almond, and add:

2 drops neroli essential oil
1 drop lemon essential oil

For relaxation
If you want to relax or sleep on a journey, try this soporific blend. Obviously, don't use it if you are driving (see page 64 for driving oils).

2 drops chamomile essential oil
1 drop lavender essential oil

Dilute in a teaspoon of carrier oil.

Mister blend for a cool journey
Dilute the following oils in one-third of a cup of water:

3 drops lavender essential oil
2 drops geranium essential oil

You can make your own portable remedies, too, by adding a few drops of neat essential oil to a handkerchief, tissue or cotton wool ball. If you are travelling in the heat, dilute the essential oils in water and keep the blend in a mister bottle to spray around your face whenever you need to cool down.

CALMING DOWN A DIFFICULT TRAVELLER

Being in a confined space with a "difficult" person usually poses a challenge. Awkward travellers can range from those who just have far too much luggage and can't help sharing it with you, to the irritating shouts-down-phone variety. Some people become irritable because they are hot or claustrophobic, whereas others just become aggressive. When you can't easily move away, dab neat lavender oil onto your wrists – the scent will calm you down and, if your fellow travellers are annoyingly close enough, this oil may soothe them, too.

AROMATIC READING

You can scent a paper or leather bookmark with essential oils for perfect, portable aromatherapy. This can be particularly helpful if you are using travelling time to work or study and need to stay alert, and also it's a pleasant way to enjoy your favourite oils as you read. Several essential oils are known to benefit concentration, specifically basil and peppermint. Sprinkle a few drops of each onto the reverse of a paper or leather bookmark (provided the back of the leather bookmark is natural and unsealed with varnish) before you set off. As the scent fades (every few days, on average), top up the bookmark with fresh oils.

Aromatherapy for driving

It's important to stay focused while driving. Regular breaks and comfortable seating, particularly on long journeys, are important; remember to stretch your arms up above your head to release tension in your hips and spine, and rotate your shoulders, wrists, and ankles. Exercise also boosts your circulation – by improving the blood flow to the brain, you also benefit from better concentration when you get back behind the wheel.

Fresh, minty oils, such as eucalyptus and peppermint, or lemon and bergamot, are recommended for driving as they are energizing and can help concentration. You can add a few drops of essential oil to tissues or cotton wool balls and leave them on the back shelf or in the side pockets of your car (see the recipes right). If these scents feel too sharp or clinical, try uplifting bergamot or lemon for a fruitier fragrance.

CAR FRESHENER
For a fresh aroma in the car, add the following blends to cotton wool balls or tissues:

2 drops peppermint essential oil
2 drops eucalyptus essential oil

Or

1 drop pine essential oil
1 drop tea tree essential oil
1 drop lemon essential oil

Or

2 drops lemon essential oil
2 drops bergamot essential oil

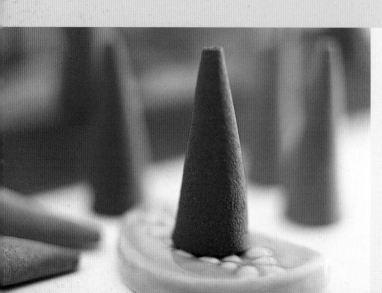

NATURAL AIR FRESHENERS
While you are away from the car, you can leave the cotton wool balls or tissues there to act as natural air fresheners, or substitute them for a sandalwood incense stick or cones. Unlit sandalwood incense gives off a sweet, mellow ambience and purifies the air.

Flying

We are much more aware of the physical effects of flying now than ever before. With DVT (deep-vein thrombosis), dehydration, and possible jet lag, it is vital to look after your health while flying to ensure that you feel well when you arrive – and can enjoy your break with energy and good spirits. Below is general advice on preventing conditions such as DVT, along with some recommended aromatherapy treatments for jet lag.

DVT ADVICE

DVT occurs when your circulation slows right down because of hours of inactivity, commonly causing blood clots in the legs, which can be fatal if they reach the heart or brain. Taking gentle, regular exercise while flying – stretching and walking up and down the aisles – keeps your circulation going and helps to prevent the formation of blood clots.

- In your seat, wiggle your toes and rotate your ankles. Push your heels into the floor then push them up to stretch the feet, ankles, and calves.
- Get up from your seat and walk around the aircraft every hour.
- If you have room, massage your knees and thighs to boost the circulation.
- Keep drinking lots of water throughout the flight to avoid dehydration.
- Wearing support socks may help.

BEATING JET LAG

Jet leg occurs when your body clock is out of sync with your surroundings – and the signs are all too familiar: exhaustion, disorientation, and frustration that you are wasting time being wide awake in the early hours.

While aromatherapy cannot "cure" jet lag, it can help to relieve some of the symptoms. Because of its direct action on the nervous system, the best oil for this is bergamot. Chamomile and lavender oils can help encourage relaxation and sleep; grapefruit, geranium, and peppermint can help stir you when you need to feel wide awake (even though it's 4am at home).

A simple way to make the most of these oils is to add chamomile and lavender oils to your bath water in the evening, and use grapefruit, geranium, and/or peppermint on a tissue so that you can inhale the invigorating aroma whenever you need an energy boost during the day. Regulating your meals so that you eat in the new time zone, and taking a few long walks can also help you to adjust your body clock.

Jet lag revival potion
On a tissue, sprinkle:

2 drops geranium essential oil
2 drops peppermint essential oil

Or

2 drops bergamot essential oil
2 drops grapefruit essential oil

And smell it throughout the day.

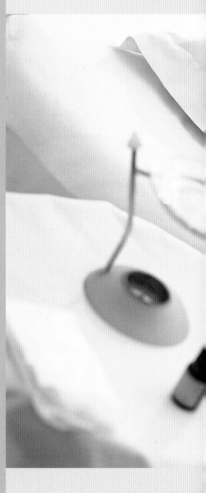

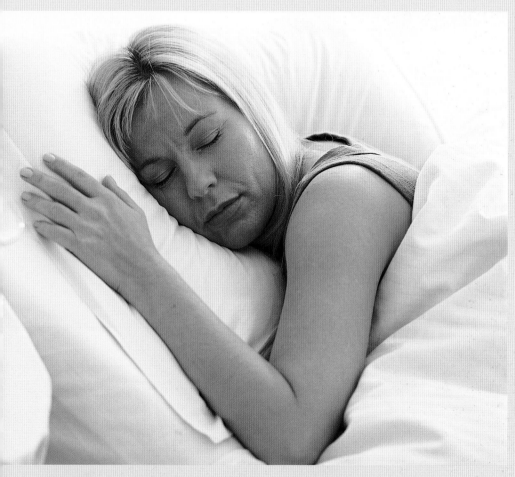

JET LAG SLEEP POTION

Run the bath and then add the following to the bath water (disperse the droplets with your hands):

3 drops chamomile essential oil
3 drops lavender essential oil

If you don't feel that you will be able to sleep, sprinkle a few drops of lavender essential oil on your pillow. You can also try drinking tea containing the herb valerian, which is readily available from health stores and many pharmacies.

Holiday aromas

On holiday we often have to deal with minor problems that don't crop up in the rest of the year, particularly if travelling overseas. Treating insect bites, nettle stings, and sunburn while keeping mosquitoes at bay, however, can almost become a way of life for a few weeks as we do battle with unfamiliar bugs and testing climates. Here are some holiday essentials:

HOLIDAY TRAVEL KIT
- Lemon (or citronella) essential oil
- Chamomile essential oil
- Lavender essential oil
- Peppermint essential oil
- Tea tree essential oil
- Thyme essential oil

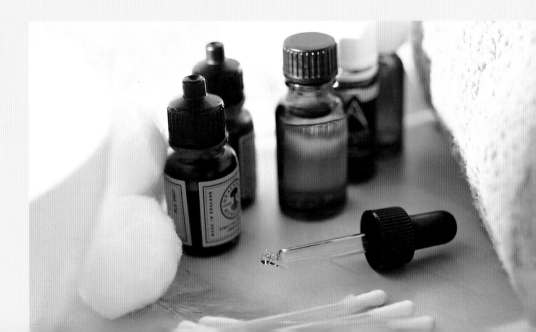

INSECT BITES
Treat with neat lavender – use a Q-tip, or cotton bud, to dab the oil directly on the bite.

STINGS
Use a cool compress to relieve stings. Soak a flannel in cool water to which you have added two drops of lemon or chamomile essential oil, squeeze the flannel out, and apply it to the sting.

INSECT REPELLENT
Preparing an insect repellent blend before you travel means you will have instant protection against those little biting bugs – and you won't smell like a dispensary either. Make a blend of the following oils, diluting them in 30ml (2 tablespoons) of carrier oil:

2 drops lavender essential oil
1 drop peppermint essential oil
1 drop lemon essential oil

Massage into exposed skin, particularly around the wrists and ankles. Alternatively, buy an essential oil or herbal insect repellent that contains neem oil. You can also burn citronella, thyme, lavender, or peppermint in an aromatherapy burner, or use citronella candles to deter mosquitoes and other undesirables.

BLISTERS (FROM FOOTWEAR)
You can use lavender and tea tree neat to treat blisters – use 1 drop of each and dab directly on the blister.

SUNBURN

Apply cold water to the burned areas first – use a flannel as a cold compress (add 3 drops lavender oil to 1 cup water) or immerse in a cool or cold bath (add 5 drops lavender essential oil to the water). When the sunburn has cooled, you can also apply a blend of lavender and chamomile essential oils, diluted in 30ml (2 tablespoons) of aloe vera gel – mix well and apply.

3 drops lavender essential oil
1 drop chamomile essential oil

Stay out of the sun until the sunburn heals, while drinking plenty of water and avoiding alcohol. Also, remember that you should not apply some essential oils to your skin before going out in the sun – an easy mistake to make if you have a massage on holiday and then want to sunbathe afterward. Check that the masseur does not intend to use bergamot, orange, grapefruit, or lemon grass essential oils. If so, you will need to cover up for 4–6 hours, otherwise the oils may irritate your skin when exposed to the sun (see the safety guidelines on pages 8–9).

HOLIDAY AILMENTS

And what are the two ailments you really don't need on holiday? Cystitis and thrush – those twin harbingers of maximum discomfort. They can be more common than usual when away from home due to the change in the water and temperature and not drinking sufficient fluids in the heat – you may find, for example, that you suffer from cystitis only when on holiday. If you need some rapid relief before embarking on the quest to find the local chemist, the following oils can help relieve some of the symptoms:

For cystitis

Sandalwood, bergamot, lavender, and tea tree can all help to treat cystitis. Add 5 drops of one of these oils to a cool bath – do not use soap or bubble bath. If you only have access to a shower on holiday, buy a large plastic bowl and have a sitz bath – add the oils to cool water in the bowl and then sit in it.

Drink plenty of water to flush out the infection and avoid alcohol. Also, look out for tea tree pessaries, which you can use to treat both cystitis and thrush.

For thrush (candida)

Try lavender or tea tree essential oils to ease the symptoms of thrush – as for cystitis, add 5 drops to your bath water. These oils act to restore natural balance to the body, and their antiseptic qualities can help banish candida albicans, the fungus that is responsible for thrush.

DIARRHOEA

If the diarrhoea is caused by nerves or bad food, make up the following blend using 30ml (2 tablespoons) of carrier oil and massage gently over the stomach:

1 drop ginger
1 drop chamomile

If the diarrhoea is caused by a virus, add 1 drop of thyme essential oil to the blend. If the condition persists, see a doctor.

CHAPTER FOUR

Aromatherapy at work

Work may be an office, your home, or outdoors, but no matter where you work, aromatherapy can make a real difference. From paper cuts to toothache, lethargy to tension headaches, essential oils can help heal physical ailments and support you emotionally throughout the day.

Most offices are charged with environmental tension. Wall-to-wall computers, air conditioning, and a lack of natural daylight contribute to a truly synthetic – and static – environment over which we have little control. Simply opening a window disrupts the office ecosystem; our glass-box workspaces are designed to circulate recycled air and dispense artificial light. All of this creates electromagnetic stress and, as our minds are preoccupied with the task in hand, our bodies are left with the job of fighting hard to cope with its effects: restlessness, anxiety, headaches, and more. Add to this the need to produce results on time and it is not so surprising that stress absenteeism, and "presentee-ism", or low productivity, are now becoming recognized as a serious challenge in many sectors as millions of working days are lost each year.

Interacting closely with others can also compromise your immunity, particularly if you are stressed out. Stress symptoms burn up your body's nutrients, leaving the immune system vulnerable and making it more likely that you will come down with coughs and colds. Essential oils can give you an energy boost, strengthen your immunity, and help you to manage unavoidable stress – and they are easy to use on the spot. You'll only need cotton wool, a few tissues, a cup, and some hot water.

Dealing with stress

Learning to identify the source of the stress around you is the first step in recognizing and managing the way you respond to your environment.

Stress can be caused by the working environment – electromagnetic stress (see page 79) can trigger tension; long hours at computer screens and substandard seating place your body under physical stress, which can be experienced as back and neck pain and repetitive strain injury (RSI), often in the shoulder, elbow, and wrist (see page 80) if using a computer for long hours. Stress can be dietary, too – a mid-morning dip in energy, for example, is often the body's stress response to you having skipped breakfast. And how we deal with stress may also be governed by behavioural patterns related to a tendency toward perfectionism or workaholism.

However, many of us identify stress as a mental process. Stress is most certainly in the mind, and it is often summoned up when we "live in the future", anticipating problems rather than seeing them as challenges or opportunities. In turn, this anxiety causes physical tension in the body, which may lead to aches and pains and other physical stress responses, such as headaches. And so the cycle continues; the mind and body, so intrinsically linked, constantly mirroring one another.

Because essential oils work holistically, treating mind and body simultaneously, they can be used to help break this stress cycle. When you choose an essential oil you can do so on the basis of its therapeutic benefit for your body and your emotions.

There are oils known for their ability to help you deal with all the different stresses you are likely to encounter during the day.

GENERAL WORKPLACE ADVICE

■ Start with the basics: insist on a comfortable, supportive chair and table adjusted to the right height. Your computer monitor should be at eye level to prevent neck and back strain. Use a gel rest at the base of the keyboard to support your wrists.

■ If you suffer regularly from headaches at work, consult your doctor; also, have your eyes tested every few years, particularly if your work involves lots of close reading, either on- or off-screen, as eyestrain may often be the culprit.

■ Take a break every hour if you are working constantly on a computer. It's hard to discipline yourself to do this, but it's vital for your physical wellbeing and will also help your concentration. Walk around, make a drink or a phone call. Stretch out your arms above your head, then to the front. Rotate your shoulders, wrists, and ankles, and gently move your head from side to side. If you suffer from back stiffness, see the exercise and recommended essential oils on pages 76–8.

■ Some people place fluorite or smoky quartz crystals on their desks to help protect them against electromagnetic stress, as they are thought to draw off negative energies.

Treating back and neck stiffness

You can help to ease back stiffness with the following exercises. Essential oils can help, but it's more effective to massage a blend into the stiff areas of the back and neck, which may be difficult to do at the office, rather than use an inhalation. Here are two blends to try:

Morning blend
Dilute in 30ml (2 tablespoons) of carrier oil:
2 drops rosemary essential oil
2 drops ginger essential oil

Evening blend
Dilute in 30ml (2 tablespoons) of carrier oil:
2 drops bergamot essential oil
2 drops lavender essential oil

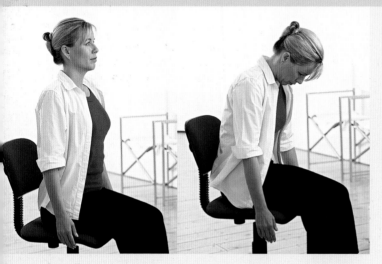

CHEST LIFT AND DIP
(01) Sit on a stool or on a chair that allows easy movement and your arms to hang naturally by your sides. Plant your feet firmly on the floor. Move your chest upward, lifting up your breast bone.

(02) Then relax and let it sink down once more. Repeat this three or four times, or as many times as are comfortable.

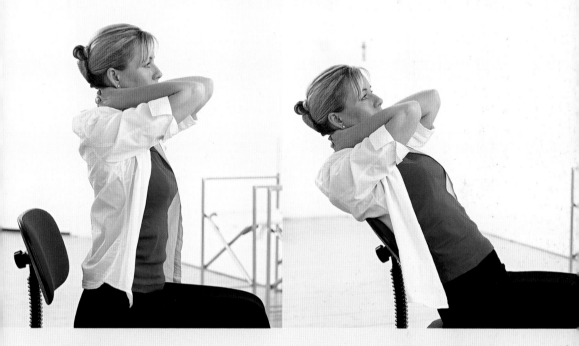

NECK CLASP

(01) Use a chair with a backrest that comes up to your shoulder blades, allowing you to lean back. Sit comfortably and rest your clasped hands behind your neck.

(02) Lean back in your chair, extending the upper part of your spine backward over the edge of the chair. Repeat this three or four times, or as many times as is comfortable.

TAKE NOTE

Practise all the movements here, and those on the following page, gently, slowly, and with concentrated awareness in order to obtain maximum benefit and to safeguard against making the muscles even tighter.

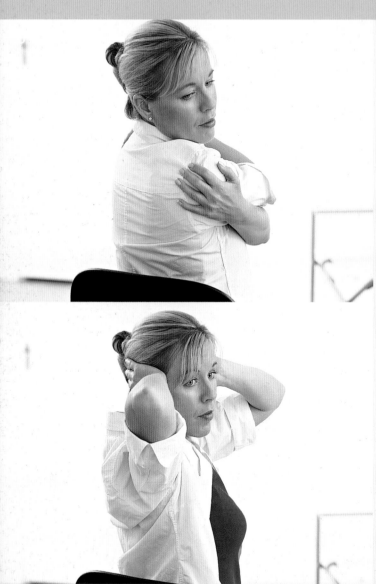

SHOULDER HOLD

(01) Sit on a stool or on a chair that allows you easy movement. Rest your feet firmly on the floor.

(02) Cross your arms over your chest. With your hands resting on your shoulders, rotate your upper trunk gently to the left, then repeat in the opposite direction. Do not over-extend. Repeat three or four times, or as many times as is comfortable.

(03) Repeat the movement, but this time with your arms straight out in front of you, with elbows at shoulder height, and again with your hands covering your ears.
  Be aware of your lower back, and take particular care not to overstretch or to pull too hard.

TREE ENERGY FOR ELECTROMAGNETIC STRESS

Many of the essential oils associated with harmonizing the effects of electromagnetic stress listed below come from trees, so in using these oils you are inviting the refreshing energy of the forest into your workspace:

- Lemon
- Orange
- Pine
- Bergamot
- Cedarwood
- Sandalwood
- Grapefruit

APPLICATIONS

Add 2 drops of your chosen essential oil to the middle of a cotton wool ball, then close the ball around it and place it behind a warm radiator. Alternatively, add 2 drops of oil to a small bowl of hot water and leave somewhere it will not be disturbed. Another option is to try an aromatherapy stone. Drop the required amount of essential oil onto the stone, which plugs into an electrical socket. This keeps the stone constantly warm so it releases a steady amount of aroma from the oils impregnated in it.

ESSENTIAL OILS FOR KICKING THE HABIT

Here is an effective essential oil treatment for tobacco or caffeine withdrawal. Dilute the oils in 30 ml (2 tablespoons) of carrier oil, and massage your wrists and temples (when at work) or your body (after a bath or shower at home). Use the blend every morning for one week to help beat the withdrawal cravings.

2 drops grapefruit essential oil
1 drop juniper essential oil
1 drop bergamot essential oil

Helping RSI

RSI, or repetitive strain injury, describes a condition that arises from repeatedly overusing the same group of muscles and joints. Habitual tasks such as painting, typing, or carrying heavy bags can, over time, cause damage to the areas under strain, resulting in RSI – a typically painful condition that is fast becoming a common complaint in the office. At the first signs of soreness or pain, seek professional help from your doctor and/or a physiotherapist. Rest your arm as much as possible. In the first instance, massage is not advisable, but gently stroking with an anti-inflammatory oil blend can help enormously. Acupuncture may also relieve RSI, as can a visit to a professional aromatherapist for a body massage – this can help RSI symptoms even when the affected areas themselves are too inflamed to be massaged. This blend uses lavender to reduce the inflammation.

RSI blend
Stroke the affected areas with this blend – do not massage:

2 drops lavender essential oil
2 drops chamomile essential oil
Dilute in 30ml (2 tablespoons) carrier oil.

Remember to seek professional advice regarding your workstation and posture, and invest in a gel pad for your keyboard if your RSI (or potential for it) may be caused by constant computer work.

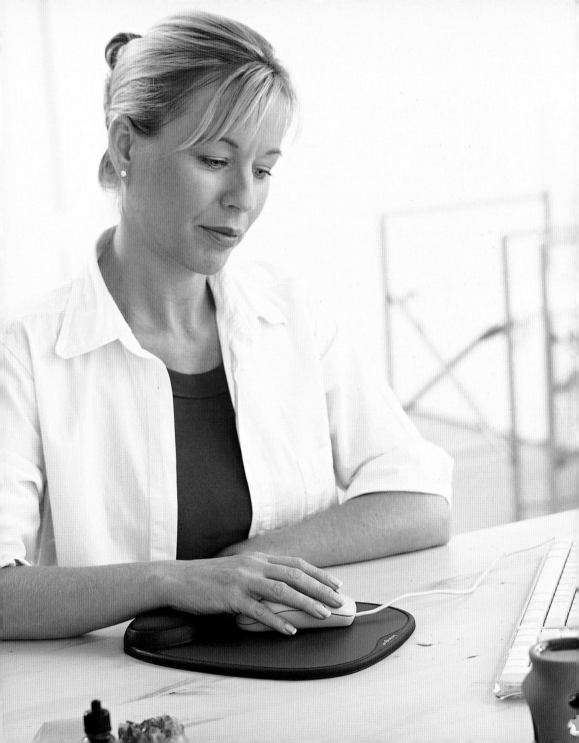

Creating an atmosphere for success

In Native American tradition, scent was used in "smudging" rituals to cure the sick and to cleanse and harmonize the atmosphere. Herbs including sweetgrass, juniper, and sage were rolled and burned, their pungent smoke wafted over the patient or into the niches of an afflicted space to purify negativity. The herbs were also burned in ritual offerings to help connect with the divine. While smudging an office isn't exactly a practicable proposition, you can still use the principles of Native American space-clearing to lift heavy energy and bring the benefit of a sweeter relationship with your colleagues.

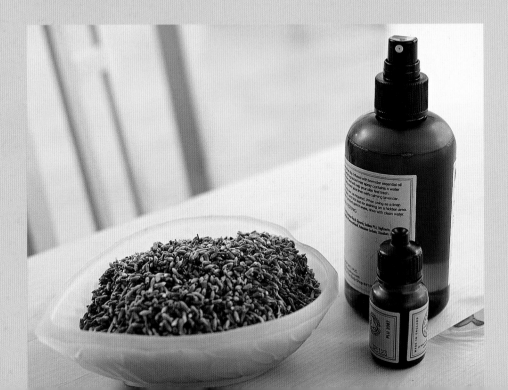

TO CLEAR THE AIR AFTER A MEETING

Sage is the staple herb in most smudge sticks, described by Nicholas Culpeper, the famous seventeenth-century physician, as good for "the lethargy [and] lowness of spirits". The essential oil from clary sage, which is a variety of sage originating around the Mediterranean, harnesses the essence of the plant so you can use it at work literally to clear the air. This room spray formula also uses pine essential oil, which is great for purifying lingering negativity. Add the essential oils below to water in a mister bottle and walk around the room spraying it into the centre of the room and into all the corners:

2 drops clary sage essential oil
2 drops pine essential oil

Use this room spray to treat an office or meeting room after a long-winded meeting, to clear that aura of tedium or tension that hangs in the air long after the participants have departed. Misting also ionizes the atmosphere, reducing the effect of static caused by electrical equipment. We experience an ionized atmosphere as a tingling invigoration from being close to, say, fast-moving water from a waterfall or fountain.

TO CLEAR THE AIR AFTER AN ARGUMENT

Juniper can help to purify any space in which the walls have probably witnessed more argument, negotiation, or criticism than you would ever be likely to hear in a lifetime. Used to encourage psychic powers by shamans, the oil may also help to stimulate your intuition – never a bad thing if you ever find yourself in an emotional minefield. The combination of clary sage and juniper makes for powerful space cleansing. Add the following oils to water in a mister bottle and walk around the room, spraying into the centre of the room and into all the corners:

2 drops clary sage essential oil
2 drops juniper essential oil

FOR PEACEFUL OUTCOMES

Lavender can cleanse an atmosphere and restore the energy of a room to neutral, so try it when you have to deal with difficult people, face to face (when the aroma benefits both parties) or over the phone (when it benefits you at first, then your calm turns to charm). To prepare for a volatile meeting or phone call, make up a lavender room spray, adding a few drops of lavender essential oil to water in a mister bottle.

Some people place a peace lily by their computers, as it is thought to absorb harmful emissions and protect from electromagnetic stress. You can display this elegant plant on your desk for similar protection.

HOME OFFICE REMEDIES

Even the home office has its problems. Although happily distanced from the conventional workplace, when we work at home we naturally create a microcosm of the bigger office we once worked in – one corner with piles of files and books, never to be touched, a groaning in-tray and lots of pens that don't

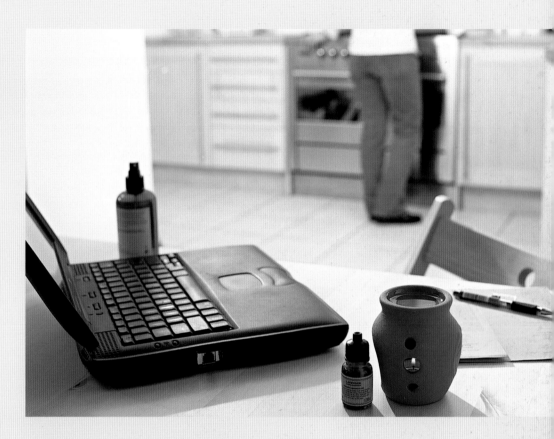

work. Also, you may have less space to work in, and the TV remote can be all too close to hand for those dull moments during the day.

To stay focused, burn basil oil in your burner (see also pages 24–7) and mist with bergamot oil to keep the energy of your home office balanced. If you live with others, lavender will help to reset the vibe to neutral so that you can shift from domestic to work mode more easily each morning.

Finding focus and energy

There is good evidence that using aromatherapy essential oils seems to help improve concentration levels while at work. Takasago, a major Japanese fragrance producer, conducted experiments into the effects of some aromas on a "typical" workforce. When lemon was pumped into the air-conditioning system, there were 54 per cent fewer typing errors.

Oils, such as basil, rosemary, and peppermint, also have a good reputation for improving concentration. So, along with the usual need to stay alert and focused while at work, these oils will also help you when your performance is under particular scrutiny. If you have examinations looming, a driving test, interview, or any situation where all your faculties must be functioning at their very best, try smelling one of these concentrated oils straight from the bottle (see page 25 for how to do this safely), or add a few drops to a tissue you can carry around, smelling the oil whenever you need a boost. This is a far better option than getting wired on strong coffee, which is more likely to cause agitation rather than relaxed focus.

ARE YOU A HOT OR COLD TYPE?

Ginger and peppermint oils are both good for dealing with the feelings of fatigue that come from prolonged stress and overwork. Ginger essential oil is more appropriate for a person who tends to feel the cold more, because the oil has a warming action on the body, whereas the cooling action of peppermint essential oil better suits those more likely to feel the heat.

OILS FOR CONCENTRATION

Essential oil	Additional benefit
Basil	Helps strengthen willpower
Lemon	May improve sense of humour
Rosemary	Boosts the memory
Peppermint	Inspires positive thinking

TEAS AND SNACKS FOR A MID-MORNING MIND BOOST

Don't forget that you can improve your mental focus by eating healthy snacks and drinking herbal teas. If you feel in need of a mid-morning boost, try the following suggestions.

Drinks
- Peppermint tea
- Hot lemon (1 slice lemon infused in hot water with an optional half teaspoon of honey; add a clove and fresh ginger root if you have a cold)
- Green tea

Snack
- A handful of sunflower seeds and linseed (flaxseed) – these are full of omega-3 and omega-6 essential fatty acids, vital for good brain function. You can also add pumpkin seeds to the mix, which is another source of omega-3 essential fatty acids.
- A few brazil nuts and dried apricots are a good source of iron.

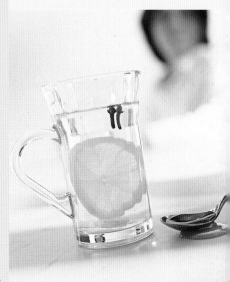

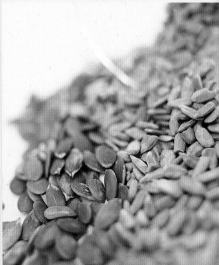

Avoiding the post-lunch dip

Post-lunch can be the lowest energy point of the day. You have eaten your midday meal and felt marginally better, but now the thought of a nap is far more appealing than working on the next quarter's production targets. Someone opens a packet of biscuits, you reach out for one, and enjoy the sweet high for all of 10 minutes before plummeting back down to your blood-sugar low. While aromatherapy can boost concentration to help improve your performance and confidence at work, it can't work effectively against a carb-fest. Go easy on too many stodgy foods, such as white pasta and bread, and opt

TO PREVENT COMFORT EATING
1 drop grapefruit essential oil
1 drop juniper essential oil
2 drops frankincense essential oil
Add to 30 ml (2 tablespoons) carrier oil and massage into your temples, wrists, and feet.

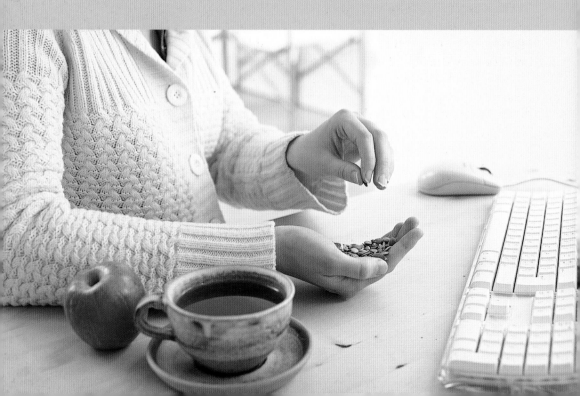

for wholemeal bread – just a single slice in an open sandwich – with fresh salads. Include fruit and vegetables to help give you energy and remember not to drink too much coffee early in the day.

If you suffer from indigestion, or want to avoid it, stop working when you eat – don't pop your food to one side of your desk and nibble as you read or tap at your keyboard. If you focus exclusively on eating, your brain knows you are eating and can activate the digestive process more effectively. This also gives you a longer food experience, making you less hungry later in the day. After your meal, have a cup of ginger tea to help digestion. You can also make your own mint tea (see below), which is delicious at any time of day – in the morning, after lunch, or when you have finished your evening meal – as it settles the stomach and is instantly refreshing. Drinking mint tea, sucking a clove bud, or chewing parsley sweetens the breath, particularly after spicy or garlic-laden food.

Mint tea for cleansing the breath and aiding digestion

Take a handful of fresh mint leaves and infuse them in a pot of boiling water. Allow the brew to sit for five minutes and then stir and mash the leaves a little to release more of the flavour. Add a half teaspoon of honey to taste, if required.

TO RELIEVE TOOTHACHE
Tooth problems often flare up when you are away from home. If this happens to you and you can't immediately get to a dentist, use a Q-tip, or cotton bud, to dab a little neat clove essential oil onto the painful area of the gum and tooth.

Oils for performance success

Some aromatherapists recommend essential oils, such as eucalyptus, rosemary, and thyme, to help improve athletic performance. You can harness the value of these oils to prepare for any high-pressure situation when it is vital that you appear relaxed, confident, and competent. Some oils, such as ginger, are ideal for dealing with the nerves that can sometimes get in the way of success. Butterflies in the tummy can almost become a distraction in themselves, taking your focus away from the task in front of you just when complete concentration is required. A good performance requires your total presence – physical as well as mental. You can use the essential oils here (see right) by adding them to a tissue and gently inhaling their aroma. Do not inhale too deeply as the effect could be overwhelming, particularly if you are already feeling a little nervous.

VIRUS PROTECTION

You can't always protect your computer from viruses, but you can protect your work environment. Tea tree oil is excellent for stimulating the immune system and warding off the many viruses that can invade offices, particularly during the winter months. You can add a few drops of neat tea tree oil to an aromatic stone, a cup of hot water, or a cotton wool ball placed somewhere warm and out of the way, such as behind a radiator, or try out the immune-boosting blend on the facing page.

PERFORMANCE FORMULA
2 drops of eucalyptus, rosemary, or thyme essential oil

Add the drops of oil to a tissue and gently inhale.

FOR BUTTERFLIES IN THE TUMMY
2 drops chamomile essential oil

Add the drops to a tissue and gently inhale. Alternatively, if you are working at home or somewhere you can apply a massage oil, dilute 2 drops of ginger essential oil in 30ml (2 tablespoons) of carrier oil and massage into your tummy area.

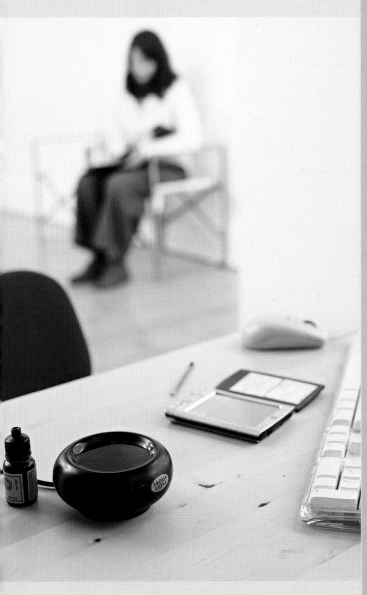

IMMUNE-BOOSTING BLEND

1 drop eucalyptus essential oil
2 drops tea tree essential oil
1 drop lemon essential oil
1 drop juniper essential oil
(you can substitute any of the above with 2 drops of pine essential oil).

Blend the oils with 30ml (2 tablespoons) carrier oil, and rub into your temples, wrists, and feet.

Helping headaches

When you are at work, headaches can result from low blood sugar levels due to hunger, dehydration – not drinking enough water throughout the day – tension, poor posture, and eyestrain, in addition to environmental factors, such as electromagnetic stress, excessive heat or cold, or poor lighting conditions. Stress can also play a major part in bringing on a headache: feeling that you just have too much to do can make your head swim. If you are affected, try the calming mini-massage (shown opposite) at your desk to relieve the distress of a headache.

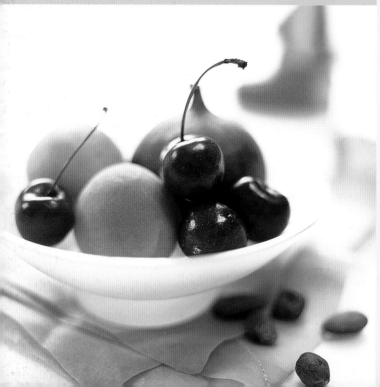

CHERRIES FOR PAIN RELIEF
Eating cherries can help the pain of a headache because they contain salicylates, which act like aspirin in the body. The fruit, a source of calcium, phosphorus, and vitamin C, is also an excellent energy booster.

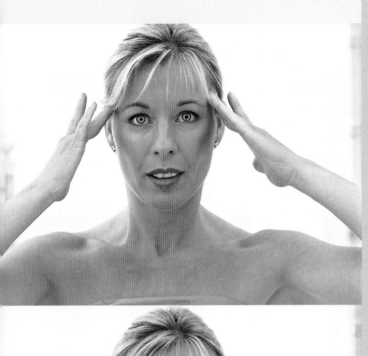

*(01) Using your middle
fingers, massage your
temples using a gentle,
circling motion.*

*(02) Gently massage around
your eyes, over the cheek
bones, and along the ridge
of the brows.*

ESSENTIAL OILS TO HELP MIGRAINE

Migraine symptoms vary from severe vision disturbances ("aura" migraines) to poor concentration, light sensitivity and/or a searing headache, sometimes down one side of the face. Stress, hormonal fluctuation, skipping a meal, or certain foods and drinks, such as red wine, coffee, cheese, oranges, or chocolate, are reported culprits. Some sufferers say that staring at a computer screen for long periods, neck tension, and tiredness can all be contributory factors. Dehydration, too, may be a cause of headaches and migraines, so remember to drink plenty of water throughout the day. If you suffer from migraines regularly, consult your doctor, medical herbalist, or professional aromatherapist.

MIGRAINE MASSAGE OIL

2 drops bergamot essential oil
2 drops chamomile essential oil
Dilute in 30ml (2 tablespoons) carrier oil and massage into your temples.

MIGRAINE COMPRESS

To a bowl of tepid water, add:
2 drops bergamot or 2 drops chamomile essential oil

Soak a flannel or a soft piece of cloth, such as a scarf, in the water, squeeze it out, and apply the compress to your forehead, as shown far right.

TREATING EARACHE
Take a small ball of cotton wool, open it out to make a dip in the centre and add 1 drop of chamomile essential oil. Close the ball and place it in your ear to relieve the pain. Make sure that the oil stays within the ball and doesn't contact any part of the ear. If the cotton wool ball is too large, simply tear off a piece to fit.

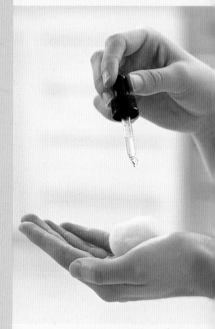

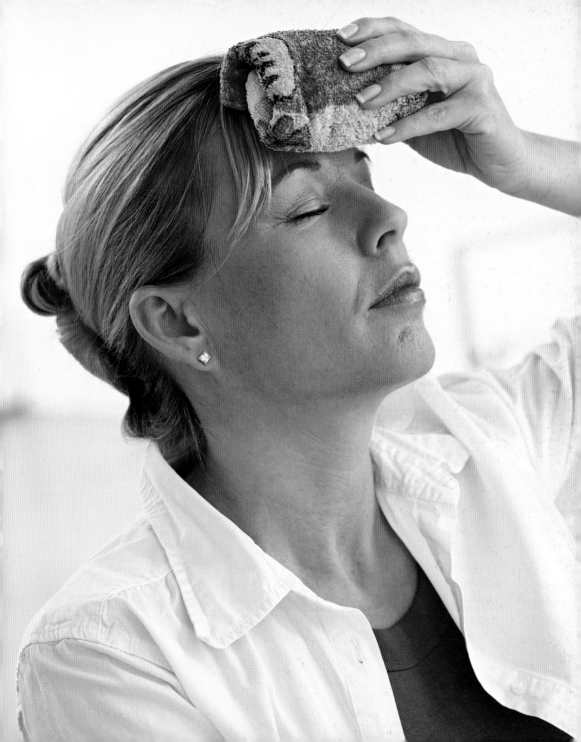

Period pains and PMS

PMS (premenstrual syndrome) is an umbrella term for a collection of premenstrual symptoms that are unique to every woman. These symptoms, which are caused by an imbalance in the hormones progesterone and oestrogen (although natural at this point in the monthly cycle) include fluid retention, tender breasts, spots, headaches, irritability, and weepiness. Some women say that their co-ordination also becomes impaired for a few days before their period commences, resulting in occasional clumsiness, and speech may be temporarily affected, with words becoming jumbled. PMS may also act as an amplifier for any existing conditions, as both physical and emotional sensitivity increases. Women can also become more sensitive to any type of pain before a period commences, and some experience extreme feelings with small problems or annoyances being blown out of proportion.

If you suffer from PMS, here are some practical guidelines that may help to alleviate symptoms:

- Take vitamin B6 or evening primrose oil to help support your cycle.
- Consider taking a magnesium supplement. Chocolate contains magnesium, which is one of the reasons women crave it before a period (as well as its sugar content). You could also try eating more calcium-rich foods, such as apricots, peaches, and almonds. If you just can't resist the chocolate option, try to choose an organic chocolate with 70 per cent or more cocoa content.

■ Avoid alcohol – some women find that they become extra sensitive to alcohol for a few days before their period starts, when drinking even a little alcohol may cause an extreme reaction.

ESSENTIAL OILS FOR PMS

Roman chamomile, geranium, lavender, bergamot, and clary sage are all helpful for PMS. Sprinkle a few drops of one of these oils onto a tissue and smell whenever you need to feel more grounded and relaxed, or inhale their aroma from a mug of hot water.

THE WISDOM OF PMS

Being premenstrual can bring the benefit of inner wisdom, a heightened awareness that helps us to identify issues often neglected or buried under the demands of a busy life. Women can also become more intuitive before a period and dream intensely, or even have prophetic dreams – another source of information and self-knowledge.

Some premenstrual women experience a burst of energy, resulting in an urge to do housework and put things in their proper place. The desire to clear things away at this time of the month mirrors the body's inner cycle – the natural flow of life – as a period is anticipated. Focusing on domestic chores may also be subconscious preparation for the first few days of bleeding, when we may feel physically below par and less able or inclined to cook and clean.

INSTANT ANTISEPTIC

At work, the classic minor accident is a paper cut, which may be more likely to occur when you are premenstrual and your co-ordination is out of kilter. To treat a paper cut with essential oils, make a natural antiseptic formula by adding a drop of lavender or tea tree oil to warm water with a few pinches of salt. Alternatively, dab the cut instantly with neat lavender.

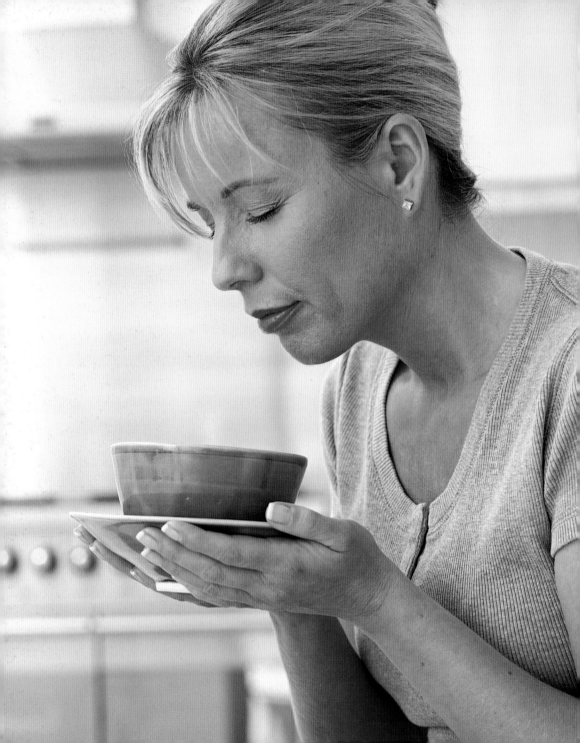

ESSENTIAL OILS FOR PAIN MANAGEMENT

Period pain varies from a low-level ache to intense cramping. The cramps are due to strong contractions of the uterus or when there is excess prostaglandin in the system. If you want to avoid using painkillers, herbal remedies can help; seek professional advice from a qualified medical herbalist.

Essential oils and herbal teas can help you deal with the initial panic or shock of intense period pain, particularly if the pain comes when you are least able to cope with it, such as when you are at work, among people you don't know, or when travelling. The most effective ways to use the following blends are as a massage mixture – dilute the essential oils in 30ml (2 tablespoons) of carrier oil – or in the bath, but at work you can inhale the oils from a tissue or from a cup of hot water to which the oils have been added (as shown left):

2 drops chamomile essential oil
2 drops ginger essential oil

Or

1 drop juniper essential oil
1 drop clary sage essential oil

Also, drink a cup of strong chamomile tea with a spoonful of honey. The sugar in the honey helps you deal with the shock of pain and the chamomile can help soothe the cramps. You can also drink chamomile tea to help with any kind of shock.

PMS ROOM SCENT

Sweetening the environment and making it more comfortable is an important form of self-nurture. Try a mister blend using the following oils diluted in water in a mister bottle:

1 drop chamomile essential oil
1 drop clary sage essential oil (not recommended for women who bleed heavily during their period)
1 drop geranium essential oil

For energy after work

Aromatherapy can help you to maintain your energy levels after work, when you want to socialize straight from the office and there is no time to go home and freshen up. The lowest point of the day for some can be around 5 or 6pm, when it's important to drink water and snack on fruit or seeds and nuts to keep your energy levels up – this is particularly important if you won't be eating a proper meal until much later in the evening. You can also use energizing essential oils that are stimulating, smell good, and keep you feeling fresh all evening.

AROMA-PERFUMES
The easiest way to use aromatherapy for an evening out is in a perfume. Choose an uplifting essential oil from the following list, add 2 drops to 1 teaspoon of carrier oil, such as almond oil, and apply to your wrists and neck:

- Geranium
- Bergamot
- Neroli
- Lemon
- Grapefruit

Keep your blend in a small, dark bottle and carry it in your handbag or briefcase, or in a bottle pendant that you can wear around your neck, and reapply the mixture as necessary.

PEPPERMINT AND BASIL TONIC
Peppermint and basil essential oils both act as brain stimulants, keeping you wakeful and alert. Use 2 drops of the peppermint and 2 drops of the basil essential oil in a mug of hot water and gently inhale the aroma. Remember, never drink essential oils, so discard the inhalation tonic after using it in case you accidentally take a sip. Alternatively, make fresh mint tea (see page 89) with half a teaspoon of honey to taste.

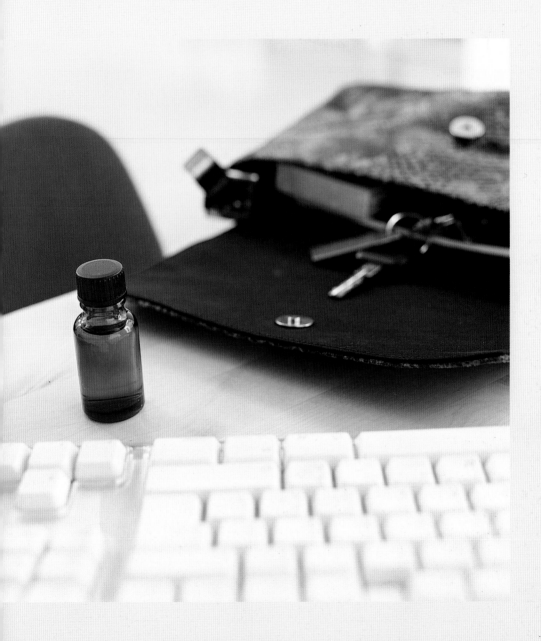

CHAPTER FIVE

Unwinding with aromatherapy

Truly unwinding means making time for yourself, time when you can fully relax. With aromatherapy you can easily treat yourself at home to enjoyable facials, massages, and luxurious baths to de-stress yourself both physically and emotionally.

Even if you have only a few hours each day to yourself, or just one evening a week in which to soothe body and soul, it's all the more vital to make the very best of the time you do have by planning your treatments in advance. And by using essential oils you know that you will be doing more than simply relaxing, because the treatments can help replenish you on a level much deeper than can be reached by slumping in front of the television or drinking a glass or two of wine.

Included in this chapter are ways to protect your skin from daily stress and regain a healthy complexion. You can also treat cellulite, or simply choose to slip into an aromatherapy bath using soporific oils, such as lavender or sandalwood, to help you de-stress. Some oils, such as rose, have both sensuous and spiritual qualities – in some traditions, anointing the heart chakra with rose essential oil before meditating was thought to help participants learn the manifestation of all kinds of love. In Eastern cultures, ylang ylang flowers were used to decorate the marital bed because they symbolized romantic love.

When you take time for yourself, you are also making time for your creativity and committing to a better work-life balance. And to achieve this, you need only your oils and a few basic massage techniques.

Aroma-facial

The following 10-minute massage will de-stress your facial muscles and help stave off the onset of fine lines and wrinkles, leaving your skin feeling rejuvenated, soft, and supple. Massage boosts circulation and helps the body to release and eliminate toxins, which can be responsible for dull skin and dark shadows. Supplement your facials with eight glasses of water a day and the most sleep you can manage, and your skin can begin to look brighter – and younger.

Essential oils are very powerful, so never use them neat. One exception, however, is lavender oil and, in some cases, tea tree.

CARRIER OILS
First, choose a carrier, or base, oil according to your skin type (see also page 139), such as:

Grapeseed oil for normal and combination skin. Sweet almond oil for all skin types, but particularly normal-to-dry skin.

To 15ml (1 tablespoon) of the base oil, add the following essential oils:

1 drop neroli essential oil
1 drop lavender essential oil
1 drop geranium essential oil

01/02

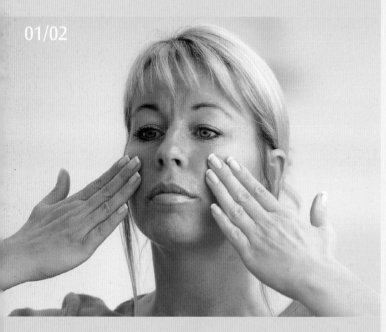

FACIAL STEPS

(01) Cleanse your face of make-up, then rinse and pat your skin dry. Ensure that your hair is pinned back from your face.

(02) Pour your oil blend (base oil with added essential oils) into the palms of your hands to warm the it. Now gently sweep both palms upward, over your face, to spread the oil evenly over your skin, avoiding the eye area. Sweep both palms upward, over your forehead.

(03) Stimulate the circulation by tapping from your chin along your jawline using your fingertips.

(04) Move up the sides of your face to your cheekbones, and tap gently along and up to the centre of the cheekbones under the eye area. Now massage under and along your cheekbones, out toward the temples. This motion helps to eliminate toxins.

(05) Gently massage both temples, using your middle and ring fingers.

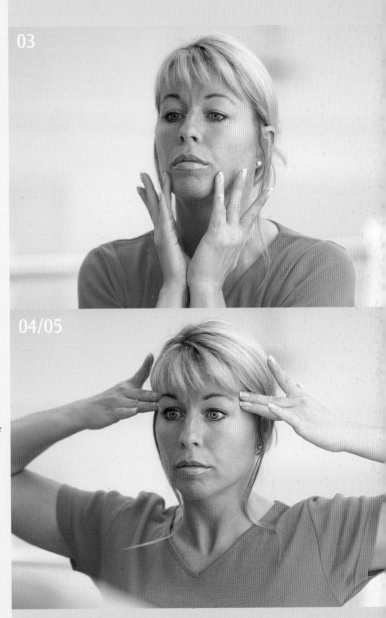

06

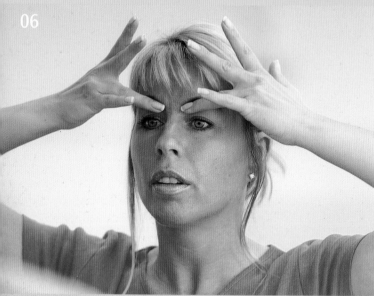

07/08

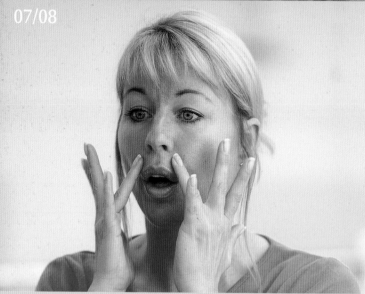

(06) Press between your eyebrows with your ring fingers, then circle the eye area by applying soft pressure at the inner eyebrow, then gliding along the eyebrow and the top of the cheekbones to the sides of your nose. Do this slowly, four or five times, to gently stimulate the skin.

(07) Now release the tension around your chin and mouth. Start by using your ring fingers to massage in small circles around your chin, and then make an "O" shape with your lips and massage upward, along the smile lines.

(08) When you have finished massaging, remove any excess oil with a tissue, but, unless you have an oily complexion, don't cleanse – let the essential oils smooth and soften your skin as you sleep. Sip water at room temperature or have a cup of herbal tea to help flush out the toxins that have been released during the massage.

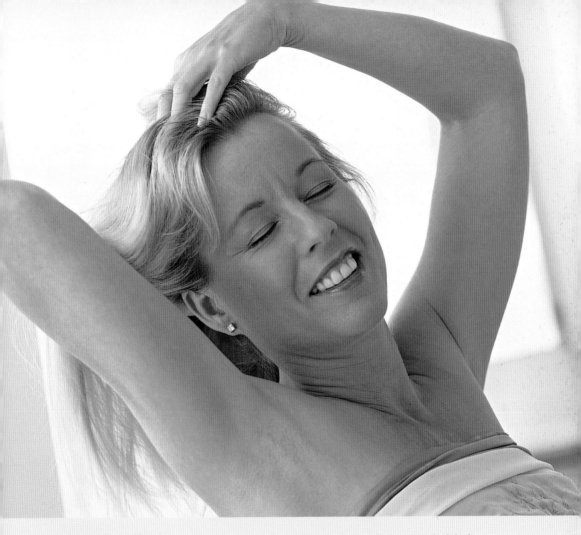

HAIR OIL

Coconut oil is renowned for making hair strong and shiny, particularly with long, normal-to-dry hair types. Use this treatment once a week. (If your hair is greasy, use almond oil and give your hair this treatment once a month). Massage a palmful of coconut oil into your hair before bed, and sleep with a towel over the pillow, or wear a shower cap over your hair if it is comfortable. In the morning, shampoo and condition as usual for glossier, deliciously scented hair.

Enhancing a youthful radiance

Many essential oils, such as those listed below, have properties to enhance a youthful radiance. When taken into the body, through an inhalation or the skin, they have an antioxidant action that slows down the ageing of the skin. Massage also stimulates the immune system and circulation, promoting the elimination of toxins. Massage oil blends are also easily absorbed into the skin, where they nourish and protect it against dryness. And carrier oils have great skin benefits, too, containing nutrients, such as vitamins A, B, and E. Aromatherapists choose them according to their clients' skin types (see page 139).

- Frankincense
- Rose
- Neroli
- Ylang ylang
- Geranium

Oil blends are best used in the evening so they can do their work as you sleep. Follow the facial massage on pages 104–6, and try this facial blend, diluting the essential oils in 15ml (1 tablespoon) of carrier oil.

1 drop ylang ylang essential oil
1 drop geranium essential oil

Or

2 drops rose essential oil

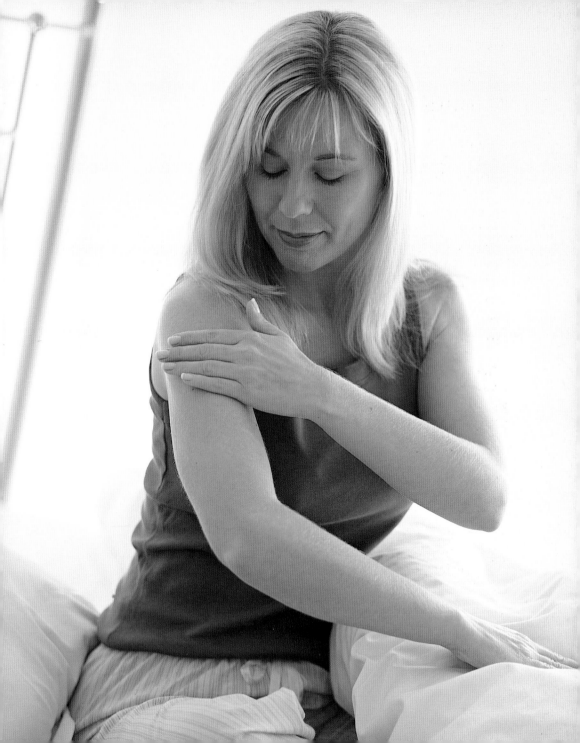

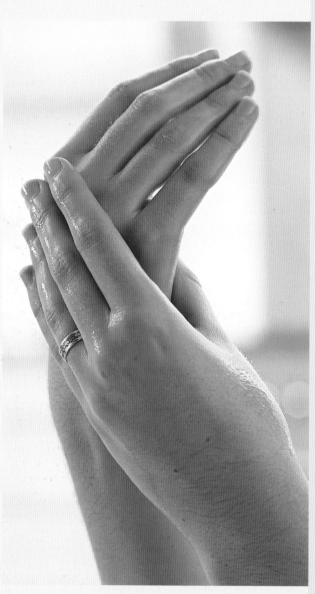

GERANIUM OIL FOR HANDS
1 teaspoon avocado oil
7.5 ml (1 dessertspoon)
almond oil
4 drops geranium essential
oil
For very dry skin, use
5 teaspoons of avocado oil
(without adding almond oil).

ANTI-CELLULITE FORMULA
Make up this body scrub in
advance:

A handful of sea salt
15ml (1 tablespoon) almond
oil, enough to make a paste
with the sea salt
2 drops grapefruit essential
oil

Wet your body and apply it
to the areas of cellulite –
typically the upper thighs
and bottom – massaging
gently with fluttery,
stimulating strokes. Shower
off the scrub, or let it melt
away in a warm bath.

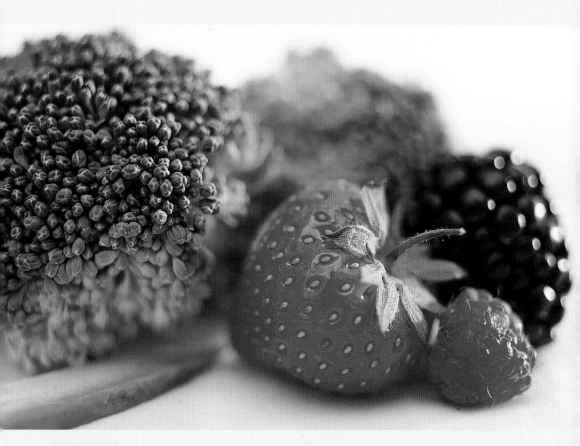

RADIANCE-BOOSTING FOODS

Certain foods are known to have an antioxidant action on the body – these include prunes, raisins, blueberries, blackberries, strawberries, raspberries, spinach, broccoli, avocado, and plums. Moderate coffee and alcohol intake, plenty of water, a healthy diet, regular exercise and a good work–life balance can also take years off your appearance.

Oils for a good night's sleep

There are many reasons for insomnia, from low blood sugar in the night to stress or mental over-activity. Using essential oils relaxes mind and body, helping to calm tension and promoting better-quality sleep. The oils principally renowned to help insomnia include:

- Lavender
- Sandalwood
- Chamomile

You might also try:

- Rose otto
- Neroli

You can make up a foot oil blend using one of the following recipes and rub it into your feet at night as an effective aid against insomnia. Frankincense calms the mind and lavender calms the emotions. Dilute in 30ml (2 tablespoons) of carrier oil:

2 drops frankincense essential oil
2 drops lavender essential oil

Or

2 drops bergamot essential oil
2 drops chamomile essential oil

Bergamot releases tensions and irritability, and chamomile instils relaxation.

INSOMNIA TIP
Some foods contain tryptophan, an amino acid that acts as a magic sleep substance. Eating a little of these foods before bed (or as a midnight snack if you can't sleep) can promote a good slumber. Try turkey, cottage cheese, or tuna on wholegrain crisp bread, or have a date, fig, or half a banana. Add lettuce to get the benefit of lactucarium, a natural sedative, or poppy seeds, which also aid sleep.

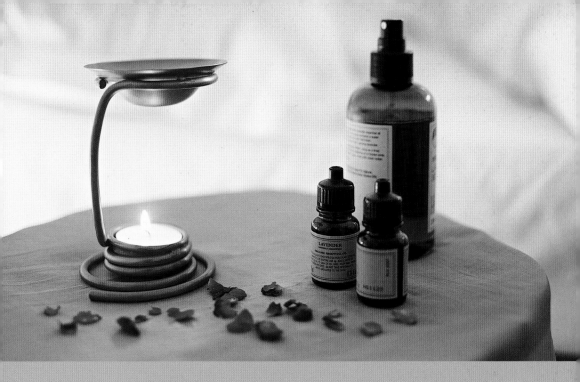

Or

2 drops rose essential oil
2 drops chamomile essential oil

Rose calms the heart; chamomile is for relaxation.

DIVINE BATHING
You can add combinations of these oils to the bathwater. Try:

2 drops lavender essential oil
1 drop chamomile essential oil
1 drop sandalwood essential oil

For a calming ambience in the bedroom, burn a little sandalwood essential oil in a burner.

SCENTING YOUR BED FOR SLEEP
Buy rosewater and decant it into a mister bottle, and spray the sheets and pillows lightly. Then you will wake up to the gorgeous sweet scent of roses.

Oils for sensuality

Scent was an intrinsic part of seduction in ancient India. The *Kama Sutra* advises a virtuous woman to wear "some sweet-smelling ointments or unguents" when approaching her husband in private, and to grow jasmine, china rose, and fragrant grasses in her garden. The ancient text *Rig Veda* mentions more than 700 substances, including cinnamon, ginger, myrrh, coriander, and sandalwood, and refers to their ritual and therapeutic uses.

   You can perfume your home with the enticing perfume of the essential oils mentioned in the blends below, or use a blend in massage. You can use the self-massage strokes on pages 30–2, or try the mini-massage, starting opposite, with a partner.

Blends for relaxed sensuality
Blend the following with 30ml (2 tablespoons) carrier oil:

2 drops lavender
2 drops geranium
1 drop ginger

Or

3 drops ylang ylang
2 drops sandalwood

Ylang ylang is an effective relaxant with aphrodisiac properties. If it is too sweet or heady for you, substitute it with jasmine.

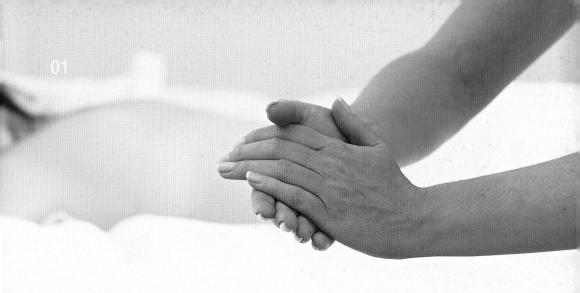

01

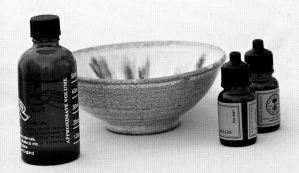

MINI-MASSAGE WITH A PARTNER

Ask your partner to lie on their stomach on the bed or on some duvets on the floor. Make sure that they are warm and comfortable. Keep the lighting low and ensure that your nails are smooth and will not snag or scratch. Remove rings or other jewellery.

(01) Kneel beside your partner with your prepared oil blend close by. Warm the oil before you start by pouring a little into your palms (do not apply straight to the skin, as it will be too cold).

(02) Begin with an effleurage stroke (see page 30), using a sweeping motion. This stroke is often used to begin or end a massage, or to connect other strokes. It's a great way to distribute the oil over the body, too, and when practised by your partner it feels very relaxing and sensuous.

(03) Cross your thumbs and rest both palms at the base of your partner's spine.

(04) Glide your hands up your partner's back. Use an even but firm pressure with your fingertips up the back, then separate your hands and sweep around and over the shoulders. Then move down the sides of the back to the waist. Practise this as one continuous, smooth stroke.

(05) Sweep your hand up and now bring them back to the starting position at the base to the spine, ready to repeat the stroke.

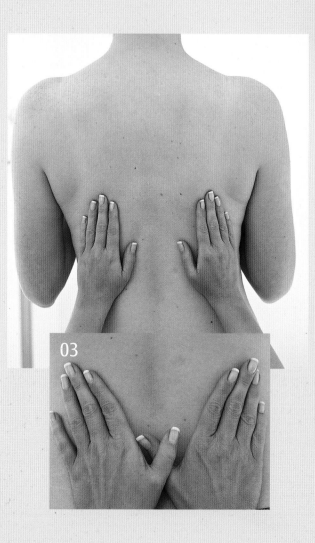

03

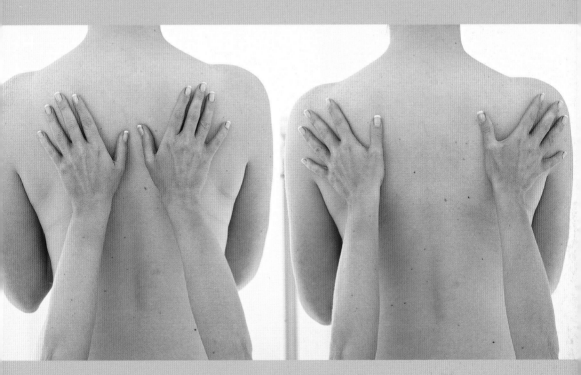

TAKE NOTE
Use your instinct and intuition while always staying
focused and gentle. Keep your hands relaxed at all
times, seeing what other movements you can use. Be
creative. You can also refer to the techniques on page
30, which you can use on different parts of the body
to complement this back massage.

CHAPTER SIX

Essential oil profiles

The first 10 oils in this chapter are those you are most likely to use every day, because they have broad emotional and physical healing applications. If you have not used essential oils before, these comprise an ideal starter kit. The 15 additional oils that follow are those you may use to extend your aromatherapy kit, when your budget allows.

Because it is vital to like the aroma of the oils you select to use, you may want to create your own top 10 favourites on the basis of their relevant healing properties, as well as their aroma. When you love the aroma of an essential oil, it can actually improve its efficacy, so use this directory as a starting point, and then follow your nose. It is thought that if an oil is the perfect remedy, it will smell beautiful to you.

The healing benefits of each of the first 10 oils are listed under headings that separate their physical benefits from their effects on the mind and spirit. Of course, the mind and body are interconnected and genuine health addresses both – so the divisions here are purely for ease of reference. The intention is to give the potential healing benefits of essential oils for common ailments, many of which are a result of daily stress.

Note also that some aromatherapy books give detailed medical benefits of essential oils for more serious conditions. See the bibliography on page 140 if you want to investigate this further.

LAVENDER *Lavendula angustifolia*

Lavender is one of the oils most commonly used to treat stress and calm the emotions. The best first-aid for burns and sunburn, lavender has one of the widest range of actions and is, therefore, a staple for the home medicine cabinet. It helps to relieve headaches and its cooling action takes the heat out of a feverish cold, so it's also vital for your bag or desk drawer. Look out for alpine lavender, which encapsulates the quiet, vast energy and space of the mountains.

The word "lavender" comes from the Latin *lavare*, to wash. The Romans added lavender to their bath water, so it is likely that the herb became synonymous with the ritual of bathing. It was also used in the birthing room to welcome the baby and soothe the mother.

Mind and spirit
This is a great oil to use if you feel overwhelmed or oversensitive; it also helps alleviate anxiety, depression, and shock. Also, lavender can be used to prepare for meditation because it balances mind and body, promoting a sense of stillness. Traditionally, the herb was used in magic rites and blessings; newlyweds were given little woven lavender wreaths to attract wealth and symbolize spiritual love.

Applications
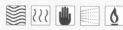
Lavender is one of the few oils that can be applied directly to the skin in small quantities to treat mild burns and bites, but it is best applied on a wet cotton-wool pad to the burn itself.

Main actions
Insomnia, migraine, respiratory infections, mild burns; an excellent anti-inflammatory.

Secondary actions
Lumbago, neuralgia, sprains, headache, cystitis, PMS, period pain, colds and flu (when feeling feverish and/or mucus is yellow), sunburn, blisters, cuts, dandruff, eczema, athlete's foot, stings, bites, spots.

Caution: Do not use lavender within the first three months of pregnancy (see pages 8–9).

CHAMOMILE *Chamaemelum nobile, Matricaria recutica*

Chamomile essential oil can be used to aid digestion and help with stomach upsets (particularly a nervous tummy), but it is perhaps best known for its ability to relieve period pain (both the essential oil, and chamomile tea, are effective; see pages 96–9), earache, and toothache. Like lavender, chamomile brings emotional balance, dispelling anxiety.

The word *chamaemelum* is from the Greek for "ground-apples", as the plant grows low and has an apple fragrance. There are two principal varieties of the herb – Roman chamomile (*Chamaemelum nobile*) and German chamomile (*Matricaria recutica*), also known as blue chamomile. Roman chamomile is best for general use, particularly for hay fever; blue chamomile has a stronger anti-viral action. The chamomile referred to in the recipes throughout this book is Roman chamomile.

Mind and spirit

Chamomile calms irritability, anger, anxiety, and depression. The principal oil used to treat children's ailments, for adults chamomile acts like a good parent, comforting the child within and alleviating the anger that arises from feeling unsupported. The plant was one of the nine sacred herbs given to the Anglo-Saxons by their god, Woden; the ancient Egyptians worshipped it for its healing properties, dedicating it to the sun god, Ra. Chamomile is also associated with protection and bringing success in all endeavours.

Applications

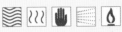

Main actions

IBS, indigestion, insomnia, period pain, hay fever, earache, nausea.

Secondary actions

Stomach upsets, neuralgia, sprains, gastro-intestinal ulcers, migraine, tension headache, toothache, PMS, eczema, boils, insect bites.

PEPPERMINT *Mentha piperita*

Peppermint is extremely beneficial when used to help settle the stomach and ease the discomfort of travel sickness. The perfect pick-me-up when your concentration and energy levels dip, peppermint, or "nature's aspirin", is also renowned for curing headaches. Peppermint is similar to chamomile in its action on the digestive system, but has a very different feel and energy – it is a stimulating oil, whereas chamomile is calming.

The word "mint" probably derives from Minthe, the nymph who, in Greco-Roman myth, was transformed into a sweet-smelling herb to be trampled underfoot.

Mind and spirit
Mint is good for treating mental fatigue and it is also associated with dispelling negative thoughts and purifying the emotions. In many countries, it was traditionally strewn on the floors of temples and homes so that when walked on the aroma was released, clearing the air.

Applications

If you mist with this oil, do not use on the face. Peppermint makes a great foot spray. In massage, use only 1 or 2 drops diluted in a carrier oil to avoid potential skin irritation. You can also add peppermint essential oil to a footbath to freshen and soothe swollen feet and/or ankles due to jet lag (see page 66) or hot weather.

Main actions
IBS, indigestion, headaches (especially tension, tiredness, and hangover headaches) nausea, pain from trapped wind, gastric flu, bad breath, travel sickness.

Secondary actions
Stomach upsets, heartburn, neuralgia, migraine, colds and flu when hot and feverish, sinusitis, swollen ankles and/or feet (due to jet lag or hot weather); makes an effective insect repellent (do not use at night, as it can keep you awake).

GERANIUM *Pelargonium graveolens*

Geranium oil is primarily a natural mood-enhancer, and it is renowned for its exquisite scent. This energizing essential oil helps to fight physical and mental fatigue, and its antiseptic properties can relieve burns, cuts, and inflamed skin.

The essential oil is distilled from several species, but the main one is *Pelargonium graveolens*, a type of rose-scented geranium that is native to South Africa. Pelargonium comes from the Greek word *palargos*, or "stork", because the fruit of the plant resembles the bill of a stork. *Graveolens* means strong or bad-smelling, which is misleading given the gorgeous scent of geranium oil. The oil from this plant has been produced for use as a perfume in Europe since the seventeenth century.

Mind and spirit
Geranium helps with anxiety and depression and is a great relaxant. Promoting a feeling of general calm, geranium is also beneficial for long- and short-term anxiety, and it works well where nervous exhaustion is due to stress and overwork. Associated with Venus, goddess of love, the geranium flower was once worn as an emblem of sexual maturity by those seeking to attract a partner.

Applications
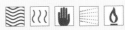

Main actions
Night sweats, hot flushes, itchy dermatitis, excessive sweating, mastitis (breast inflammation); mood-enhancer; perfect oil to treat all the symptoms stemming from the menopause.

Secondary actions
PMS, cystitis, dry skin, itching, parasitic skin conditions, boils, abscesses, psoriasis.

KEY TO SYMBOLS

 Use in bath

 Use for inhalation

 Use in massage

 Use in a mister bottle on hair or skin

 Use in an oil burner – or a diffuser or vaporizer

 Use as a perfume

BERGAMOT *Citrus bergamia*

Bergamot is a refreshing and an uplifting oil that helps to ease both physical and emotional tension. Like most therapeutic essential oils, it has antiseptic properties and it is also reputed to benefit the respiratory system.

According to many sources, bergamot was named after the Italian city of Bergamo in Lombardy, where it was first sold. Another theory is that the word bergamot is a corruption of Pergamum, a city in Asia Minor (now Turkey), or that it came from the Turkish word *beg-armundi*, meaning "Lord's pear" – a reference to the shape of the fruit. In Napoleonic times, bergamot was popularly used as a perfume. Bergamot essential oil is added to black tea in order to make Earl Grey tea.

Mind and spirit
Bergamot regulates the nervous system, relieving nervous depression and anxiety, and helps with frustration, encouraging the release of pent-up emotions. It's good to use whenever you feel "stuck" in your life, as it has a lightening and moving quality, which also helps to reduce addictive urges.

Applications

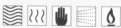

Main actions
General tension throughout the body such as tension headaches, IBS, mild asthma, or a feeling of constriction in the chest, flatulence, irritable and painful periods.

Secondary actions
Lung infections, urogenital infections such as cystitis, oily conditions such as acne and seborrhoea, flu when accompanied by irritability; heals wounds.

Caution: As with most essential oils, never use undiluted bergamot on the skin as it can irritate. Do not use even the diluted oil on the skin and then expose yourself to the sun or have laser hair removal treatments as bergamot makes the skin photosensitive (see also the safety guidelines on pages 8–9). Use as a room spray only; do not mist the face or body.

GINGER *Zingiber officinale*

Ginger is great for travel sickness, physical fatigue, and pain relief. It eases aching muscles, boosts immunity, calms the pain of rheumatism (when the onset of pain is caused by cold conditions), and helps with period pain. This healing, replenishing oil is also used to help the recovery of postnatal women; in Malaysia, women traditionally eat ginger chicken for 40 days after childbirth as a uterine tonic.

Ginger's ability to promote good digestion is legendary. The edible root is used in cooking and as a tea for its spicy flavour and cleansing effect. The word "ginger" may have come from the Gingi district in India, where the plant originated, and ginger tea was made to treat stomach upsets.

Mind and spirit
Imported into Europe during the Middle Ages, ginger has been used as a medicine and for magic rituals. It features as a prominent herb in traditional Chinese medicine, thought to bring efforts to fruition more quickly. It may heighten general sexual enjoyment due to its ability to increase energy, health, and vitality.

Applications
 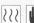

Ginger can be used for massage, taking extreme care not to exceed the dosage given in recipes. A massage blend applied directly to painful areas or a warming winter foot blend work best.

Main actions
Travel sickness, indigestion, upset stomachs (including diarrhoea, gastric flu, and abdominal swelling), respiratory infections, colds and flu, sore throat; boosts circulation and warms hands and feet; perfect winter tonic.

Secondary actions
Pain or cold in lower back, muscle tension, general rheumatic pain, painful periods.

Caution: If adding ginger essential oil to the bathwater, make sure the oil is well dispersed before getting in. Avoid ginger if you have sensitive skin.

TEA TREE *Melaleuca alternifolia*

Tea tree is one of the best-known and most frequently used of all the essential oils, because it is a brilliant infection-fighter – from fungal infections, such as athlete's foot, to severe flu, infected wounds, insect bites, and mouth ulcers.

Tea tree oil comes from Australia, including the off-shore state of Tasmania, and was used by the Aborigines; the leaves were picked and either chewed or boiled in water to make cures for colds and flu. Captain James Cook in 1770 found this sticky bush growing in Botany Bay, New South Wales, and made a herbal tea from it. This became known as "tea tree" and was a popular remedy used by early immigrants. Tea tree was recognized by the *British Medical Journal* in 1933 as a "powerful disinfectant".

Mind and spirit

Tea tree oil is best known for its physical attributes, but it also benefits the mind, as confidence is enhanced by a sense of physical wellbeing. The oil is thought to strengthen willpower and a person's sense of self-esteem.

Applications

Tea tree oil can be used neat on a cotton bud, or Q-tip, in small quantities to treat cold sores, bites, and stings. If added to your bathwater, use only 1 or 2 drops to avoid skin irritation.

Main actions

Respiratory infections such as bronchitis, laryngitis, dental abscesses; infections of the urinary tract, such as thrush, herpes, cystitis; immune booster, makes a perfect flu remedy.

Secondary actions

Acne, athlete's foot, blisters, infected wounds, dandruff, chicken pox, shingles.

BASIL *Ocimum basilicum*

Basil is an energizing herb originating in Asia and used by the Romans and in Galenic medicine. Basil is the best oil to wake up the brain and, therefore, has been used for centuries to treat nervous debility. It is also an ingredient in many restorative tonics. In Italy, the herb is used extensively in cooking not only for its wonderful flavour, but also to activate the mind and boost immunity.

Mind and spirit
Basil essential oil is great for improving concentration when burned, it certainly focuses the mind and boosts willpower. It also helps to relieve anxiety and depression, releasing worries and feelings of guilt and giving a sense of happy abandon. The herb can also be good for people who continually ponder whether or not they have done the right thing, resulting in stress and indigestion; it's a perfect remedy, too, for those who make plans but do not carry them through.

The heart-shaped leaves of the basil plant are thought to be love symbols.

Applications

Use only 1 or 2 drops to avoid skin irritation.

Main actions
Nervine tonic, brain stimulant, eases depression resulting from exhaustion, lower backache, tiredness, headache.

Secondary actions
Chronic cough or bronchitis, nasal congestion or loss of sense of smell, lung infection, especially when tired and tense.

KEY TO SYMBOLS

 Use in bath

 Use for inhalation

 Use in massage

 Use in a mister bottle on hair or skin

 Use in an oil burner – or a diffuser or vaporizer

 Use as a perfume

SANDALWOOD *Santalum album*

Sandalwood is a great oil for treating cystitis and for helping with respiratory infections. A beautifully scented oil, it calms the mind and is thought to promote a connection with the divine. This sensuous oil is also reputed to be an aphrodisiac.

Sandalwood has been, and continues to be, an integral part of everyday life in Asia, where the wood has been used for carving temples and for making furniture and religious icons.

Mind and spirit
Sandalwood can help to alleviate depression, anxiety, and insomnia because it enables you to reconnect with your essential inner-self, reminding you of who you really are inside regardless of external pressures and worldly desires. As mentioned above, it relaxes the mind and aids meditation. Sandalwood has always had associations with spiritual life, as temples were made from the tree; sandalwood incense is burned in Hindu and Buddhist rituals.

To make sandalwood perfume, don't apply the oil neat to the skin. Instead, make a blend by adding 5 drops of oil to a teaspoon of carrier oil.

Main actions
Cystitis, respiratory infections, especially those with a harsh, painful cough.

Secondary actions
Dry skin, itching, inflammation, eczema; good for hot, agitated, emotional states that lead to headaches, nervous exhaustion, or insomnia.

Applications

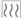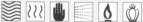

ROSEMARY *Rosemarinus officinalis*

Rosemary can sharpen your wits and enhance your memory, and it can also help to ease aches and pains and boost the circulation. Women traditionally rinsed their hair with rosemary water for clean, gleaming results.

The herb was used extensively by ancient Egyptians, Romans, and Greeks to whom it was sacred; it also symbolized friendship and loyalty. The word "rosemary" is derived from the Latin *ros marinus*, meaning "rose of the sea". First distilled in the thirteenth century, rosemary essential oil has a long history and wide range of therapeutic uses.

Mind and spirit

Rosemary can enhance memory, and it is also good for correcting apathy and mental fatigue. An exhilarating oil, it instils enthusiasm and bolsters self-confidence, restoring faith in our innate potential. As rosemary boosts the memory, it is a reminder of your true calling in life.

Applications

Use only 1 or 2 drops of oil in the bath or for massage to avoid skin irritation.

Main actions

Physical weakness and recuperation after illness; muscle stiffness and pain, especially backache, poor circulation, memory loss.

Secondary actions

Poor concentration, colds, catarrh, and bronchitis.

Caution: Do not use rosemary essential oil during pregnancy, or if you have high blood pressure or epilepsy.

KEY TO SYMBOLS

 Use in bath

 Use for inhalation

 Use in massage

 Use in a mister bottle on hair or skin

 Use in an oil burner – or a diffuser or vaporizer

 Use as a perfume

CLARY SAGE *Salvia sclarea*

Main actions
Strong action on the female reproductive system, particularly easing menstrual cramps and menopausal symptoms. Anti-depressant, brings wisdom.

Secondary actions
Sore throat, very good for stress and post-natal depression, strengthens physical and spiritual sight.

Applications

Use only 1 or 2 drops of oil in the bath or for a massage to avoid skin irritation.

Caution: do not use during pregnancy. Excessive doses may bring on epileptic fits so always use sparingly. Do not use if prone to heavy periods, as this oil promotes menstrual blood flow.

EUCALYPTUS *Eucalyptus globulus*

Main actions
Nasal congestion, sinusitis, colds and flu symptoms (especially when feeling chilled), bronchitis, and asthma.

Secondary actions
Cold sores, general infections – especially urinary and intestinal – neuralgia, insect repellent, supports the immune system, good antiseptic, general anti-inflammatory.

 Applications

Use only 1 or 2 drops of oil in the bath or for a massage to avoid skin irritation.

JUNIPER *Juniperus communis*

Main actions
Strengthens the kidneys, extremely good for general physical weakness and cold limbs, menstrual cramps (when feeling cold), and pain in lower back. Provides the energy necessary to give up bad habits and begin better ones. Removes emotional toxins.

Secondary actions
Water retention, cystitis, oily skin and scalp, coughs, cellulite, improves circulation, aids weight loss by helping you to change to healthy eating habits as well as having a diuretic action.

Applications
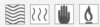

Caution: do not use during pregnancy.

LEMON *Citrus limon*

Main actions
Cooling oil that helps a wide range of infections: respiratory infection, mouth and digestive infections, skin infections, such as herpes and ringworm; good insect repellent; dissipates irritability.

Secondary actions
Bursting headaches, hangover effects (cleanses liver), cellulite, obesity, high cholesterol, gout, insect bites. Gives mental clarity and decisiveness, stimulates the left brain as well as promoting a sense of humour. Also has a unique action as a deodorant.

Applications
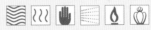

Use only 1 or 2 drops of oil in the bath or for a massage to avoid skin irritation.

NEROLI *Citrus aurantium*

Main actions
Agitation, insomnia, nervous tension, palpitations, relaxant.

Secondary actions
Dry or sensitive skin, broken capillaries, aphrodisiac (good for lack of sex drive due to tension or sadness).

Applications
   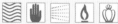

Use only 1 or 2 drops of oil in the bath or for a massage to avoid skin irritation.

PATCHOULI
Pogostemon patchouli

Main actions
Aphrodisiac (eases sexual anxiety), depression, eczema, acne, impetigo, herpes, fatigue.

Secondary actions
Loose stools, abdominal distension, inflamed or chapped skin, boosts immunity, helps you to reconnect with body and sensuality.

Applications
    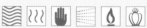

Use only 1 or 2 drops of oil in the bath or for a massage to avoid skin irritation.

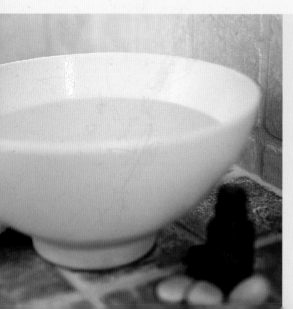

KEY TO SYMBOLS

 Use in bath

 Use for inhalation

 Use in massage

 *Use in a mister bottle on hair or skin*

 Use in an oil burner – or a diffuser or vaporizer

 Use as a perfume

FRANKINCENSE
Boswellia thurifera

Main actions
Quiets internal chatter, helps with tightness in the chest, especially good for dry cough and laryngitis, reduces heavy menstrual flow or bleeding between periods.

Secondary actions
Good for mature skin conditions – helps prevent wrinkles; helps when feeling overwhelmed by mental impressions, makes a person focused and single-minded and therefore aids meditation.

Applications
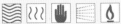

PINE *Pinus sylvestris*

Main actions
Colds and flu when feeling chilled, lethargy, sore throat, dealing with the negativity of others – helps to dispel negative energy.

Secondary actions
Loss of appetite, cystitis, water retention, gout, sinusitis, catarrh. Strong antiseptic, good for fatigue and nervous debility, brings a positive attitude, helps take away negative self-image. Can additionally be used in saunas and steam baths.

Applications
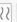

Use only 1 or 2 drops of oil in the bath or for a massage to avoid skin irritation.

ROSE OTTO
Rosa damascene; R. centifolia

Main actions
Anger, depression, insomnia, helps instil tolerance; best hangover remedy, good for a broken heart or grief, dry skin conditions; all-round remedy for female reproductive system.

Secondary actions
Boils, constipation, headache, migraine, PMS, broken capillaries, anxiety; also an aphrodisiac. In folklore, rose is thought to calm domestic strife.

Applications
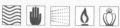

THYME *Thymus vulgaris*

Main actions
Excellent antiseptic for the intestine, gastric virus, helps sore throat, raises blood pressure. Very good expectorant.

Secondary actions
Backache, fatigue, gets rid of lice and nits, helps clear excessive emotions from the past, gives courage, helps to take a deeper breath of life.

Applications

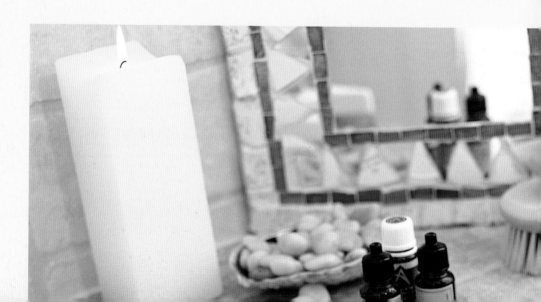

YLANG YLANG *Cananga odorata*

Main actions
Calms the heart, good for palpitations; eases tension, insomnia and depression, restores a sense of joy.

Secondary actions
Impotence, frigidity, intestinal infections (especially with fever) soothes the skin, very good for oily skin. Petals were traditionally used to decorate the beds of newly-weds.

Applications
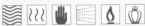

JASMINE *Jasminium officinale*

Main actions
Harmonizes the sexual and emotional aspects, regulates menstruation, eases painful labour and periods, helps diarrhoea, coughs (especially a dry cough and hoarseness), moistens the skin – good for most dry skin disorders.

Secondary actions
Depression, anxiety, helps to ease a sense of tightness in the chest, enhances feelings of love and uplifts the heart.

Applications
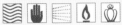

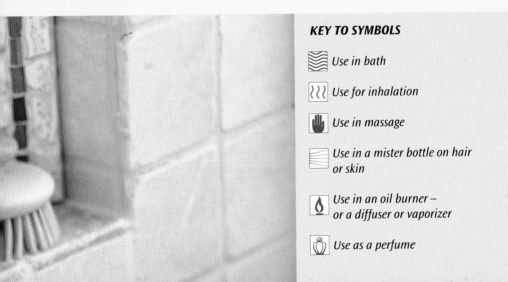

KEY TO SYMBOLS

Use in bath

Use for inhalation

Use in massage

Use in a mister bottle on hair or skin

Use in an oil burner – or a diffuser or vaporizer

Use as a perfume

GRAPEFRUIT *Citrus paradisi*

Main actions
Cellulite, obesity, constipation, feeling bad tempered; has cleansing action, mild diuretic, helps oily skin, refreshing.

Secondary actions
Stretch marks, frustration, helps with tendency to comfort eat, promotes lightness of spirit.

Applications
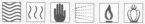

CLOVE *Eugenia caryophyllata*

Main actions
Toothache, neuralgia, upset stomach, respiratory infections; a warming winter oil.

Secondary actions
Restores appetite, helps general infections, a relaxant, helps when giving up smoking. Sucking a clove is a good antidote for garlic breath. Aphrodisiac, increases intuition.

Applications

KEY TO SYMBOLS

 Use in bath

 Use for inhalation

 Use in massage

 Use in a mister bottle on hair or skin

 Use in an oil burner – or a diffuser or vaporizer

 Use as a perfume

CEDARWOOD *Cedrus atlantica*

Main actions
Lethargy, lack of confidence, urogenital problems, cellulite, bronchitis, lower backache.

Secondary actions
Promotes tissue repair, good for oily skin, preserves a sense of identity so helps with feelings of alienation; a very grounding oil that helps a person feel settled and rooted in new surroundings.

Applications

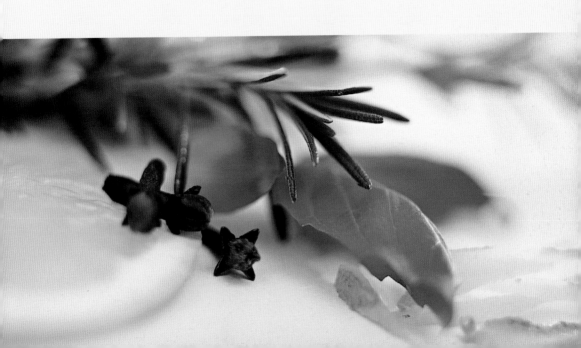

Carrier oils

Few oils can safely be applied directly to the skin straight from the bottle, so they need to be diluted in a base, or carrier, oil. The carrier oil also "fixes" an essential oil, preventing its immediate evaporation – just a drop of neat essential oil will disappear in seconds when exposed to the air.

There are various carrier oils available. The list opposite is not intended to be comprehensive, but includes those most commonly available and used.

When you make up an essential oil blend, mix the essential oils and carrier oils together in a small cup or beaker, remembering to store it in an airtight dark bottle away from sunlight to prevent deterioration.

JOJOBA OIL
The Aztecs were said to have anointed babies with jojoba oil to give their newborns lifelong health and beauty.

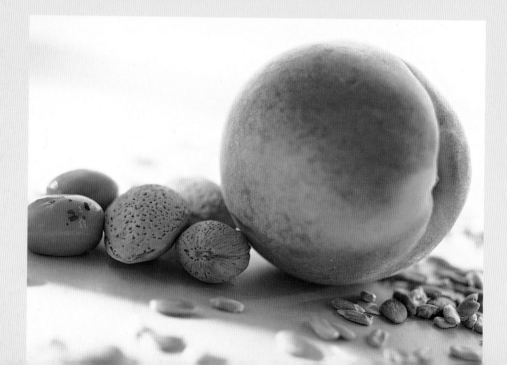

CARRIER OILS AND SKIN TYPES

Essential oil	Benefits	Texture
Sweet almond oil	All skin types	Light
Apricot kernel	All skin types	Light
Avocado	Dry and mature skin	Rich, dilute with a lighter oil, such as almond
Grapeseed	All skin types, particularly oily skin	Light
Coconut oil	Best for scalp and hair treatments, foot rubs	Light to medium
Jojoba	All skin types – balancing action helps oily and dry skin; good hair oil	Medium
Calendula	Special oil for inflamed or damaged skin, such as scarring and eczema	Rich
Wheatgerm	Dry, mature, damaged, or scarred skin.	Rich, dilute with a lighter oil, such as almond

Further reading

Aromatherapy: The Encyclopedia of Plants and Oils and How they Help You, Danièle Ryman, Piatkus, 1993

Aromatherapy for Healing the Spirit, Gabriel Mojay, Gaia Books, 1996

Culpeper's Complete Herbal, Nicholas Culpeper, Foulsham

Essential Oils, Susan Curtis, Haldane Mason, 2002

The Fragrant Pharmacy: A Complete Guide to Aromatherapy and Essential Oils, Valerie Ann Worwood, Bantam, 1991

The Illustrated Encyclopedia of Essential Oils: The Complete Guide to the Use of Oils in Aromatherapy and Herbalism, Julia Lawless, BCA/Element Books, 1995

Practical Aromatherapy: How to use Essential Oils to Restore Health and Vitality, Shirley Price, Dealerfield/ HarperCollins, 1994

Index

ACKNOWLEDGEMENTS

The author would like to thank Daphne Roubini for her valued
consultancy work on this book and, in particular, for the essential oil
recipes and directory; Jonathan Hilton and Peggy Sadler for their great
editing and design work respectively; and Jo Godfrey Wood, who
inspired it all.

Gaia Books would like to thank Caron Davis for modelling.